Local Immunotherapy in Allergy

··························

Chemical Immunology and Allergy

Vol. 82

Series Editors

Johannes Ring   Munich
Luciano Adorini   Milan
Claudia Berek   Berlin

KARGER

Local Immunotherapy in Allergy

Volume Editors

Udo R. Markert Jena
Peter Elsner Jena

18 figures, 1 in color and 22 tables, 2003

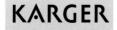

Basel · Freiburg · Paris · London · New York ·
Bangalore · Bangkok · Singapore · Tokyo · Sydney

Chemical Immunology and Allergy

Formerly published as 'Progress in Allergy' (Founded 1939),
continued 1990–2002 as 'Chemical Immunology'
Edited by Paul Kallos 1939–1988, Byron H. Waksman 1962–2002

....

Udo R. Markert

Doctor, Department of Dermatology and Allergology,
Friedrich Schiller University, Jena

Peter Elsner

Professor, Department of Dermatology and Allergology,
Friedrich Schiller University, Jena

Bibliographic Indices. This publication is listed in bibliographic services, including Current Contents® and Index Medicus.

© Copyright 2003 by S. Karger AG, P.O. Box, CH–4009 Basel (Switzerland)
www.karger.com
Printed in Switzerland on acid-free paper by Reinhardt Druck, Basel
ISSN 1660–2242
ISBN 3–8055–7531–9

....
Contents

Contents

Contents

Contents

109 Safety of Allergen-Specific Sublingual Immunotherapy and Nasal Immunotherapy

G. Passalacqua, F. Fumagalli, L. Guerra, G.W. Canonica, Genoa

Evidence Base

119 The WHO ARIA (Allergic Rhinitis and Its Impact on Asthma) Initiative

C. Bachert, P. van Cauwenberge, Ghent

Prospects for the Future

127 Local Immunotherapy in Allergy: Prospects for the Future

U.R. Markert, Jena

Contents

....

Foreword

Incidence and prevalence of allergies are an increasing phenomenon worldwide. The most efficient therapy is the avoidance of the allergen. This, unfortunately, is not practicable in most cases. Antihistamines provide a very well-acting and well-accepted symptomatic treatment, which in its recent form is liberated from most side effects and which can be easily applied locally or systemically over a long period. At present new promising and interesting methods of symptomatic treatment are available, such as antileukotrienes or anti-IgE.

The only accepted curative treatment is the immunotherapy, formerly known as hyposensitization or desensitization and recently called 'vaccine'. The subcutaneous application undoubtedly has clinical efficacy, but it displays several inconveniences, such as the need to visit a doctor for its application, its invasiveness, which many patients, especially children, do not tolerate psychologically or the rare but possible side effects. Local immunotherapies were invented to avoid these inconveniences and some forms, namely the sublingual and the nasal application, seem to accomplish this goal successfully. Regarding the clinical efficacy, opinions still widely differ. An increasing number of international placebo-controlled double-blind studies demonstrate clinical and sometimes immunological efficacy, but direct comparisons between the subcutaneous and the local routes have thus far been very poor. Studies on the long-term efficacy of local immunotherapies are also rare, because this therapy has been in clinical use for not much longer than 10 years. Local immunotherapies, furthermore, need a better or at least more transparent standardization of, for example, applied allergen concentrations, application intervals and duration, or combination therapies with different allergens or other allergy medications.

In the first part of this volume, the reader will find information concerning general aspects of immunotherapy, its history, the allergen resorption and its biodistribution as well as aspects derived from clinical experience. In the second part, the most relevant international studies on sublingual and nasal immunotherapies are reviewed, possible side effects are discussed and some new original data are provided. In the last chapter, Prospects for the Future, I will give a critical overview regarding the most unresolved and troublesome aspects of local immunotherapies and would thereby like to motivate the scientific community to intensify their efforts to investigate and ameliorate this promising branch of potentially curative antiallergy therapy.

Udo Markert, Jena

Markert UR, Elsner P (eds): Local Immunotherapy in Allergy.
Chem Immunol Allergy. Basel, Karger, 2003, vol 82, pp 1–10

······················

Local Immunotherapy in Allergy

*David L. Morris, George F. Kroker, Vijay K. Sabnis,
Mary S. Morris*

Allergy Associates of La Crosse, Ltd., La Crosse, Wisc., USA

Key Words
Sublingual immunotherapy · Subcutaneous immunotherapy · Allergy

Abstract
Specific immunotherapy is a very powerful tool which is currently underutilized in the treatment of allergies. Sublingual immunotherapy (SLIT) has many advantages over subcutaneous immunotherapy (SCIT), and has been well proven to work for many pollens and dust mites. Multiple studies have shown SLIT improves symptoms and reduces the reliance on medications. Sublingual treatment has been studied in Europe and is endorsed by the World Health Organization Committee on Immunotherapy as a viable alternative to SCIT.
Conclusion: SLIT offers another option for patients who are not currently candidates for subcutaneous immunotherapy. Because of improved safety, convenience and compliance, sublingual immunotherapy should be used as a first-line treatment option.

Specific immunotherapy is the ideal way to treat allergies. The primary goal is to desensitize the patient for the underlying cause of allergy symptoms by making them more tolerant to specific allergens. Immunotherapy is a powerful tool to decrease nasal and eye allergy symptoms as well as asthma. It is a common understanding in the allergy profession that immunotherapy is currently underutilized.

Specific immunotherapy using subcutaneous injections (SCIT) has been used for almost 100 years. It is clearly helpful for allergic rhinitis from pollens. Treatment of asthma, especially from molds, is not as clearly successful. Factors such as the inconvenience and expense of traveling for allergy shots contribute to a dropout rate greater than 50% over a multiyear course of treatment [1]. Some children and adults dislike injections or have had reactions to allergy shots.

Sublingual immunotherapy (SLIT) has many advantages over subcutaneous treatment. It has shown efficacy for allergic rhinitis and asthma due to dust mites, pollens, and molds [2–8]. Pollen studies include *Parietaria* [9–13], grass [14–21], ragweed [22], and trees [23, 24]. SLIT works for children [3, 6, 7, 17, 23] as well as adults. It can be used for food allergies to help patients develop tolerance to specific foods [25, 26]. Treatment of children with atopic dermatitis [27] or nasal allergy may even help prevent the progression to asthma.

The mechanism of action for SLIT as well as SCIT has not been fully elucidated. It has been shown that sublingual antigens stay in the mucosa for up to 20 h after administration [28]. Studies using radioactive labeled *Parietaria* delivered sublingually showed plasma levels peaked in 2 h [29]. One likely mechanism is that the sublingual antigens act on ganglionic cells (antigen-presenting cells) in the mucosa to develop tolerance to the allergens. Local 'mucosal immunity' appears to play a significant role [30]. Because sublingual swallow delivery has been more efficacious than sublingual spit, oral tolerance mechanisms in the gut may also be a factor [31, 32].

Sublingual treatment has been used for many years. Many allergists in the US (especially otolaryngic allergists) [33] use sublingual treatment for inhalant as well as food allergies. Case reports of treatment for food allergies and respiratory inhalant allergies were published in 1969 and 1970 [34, 35] in the US. In our clinic, we have treated over 60,000 patients in the past 35 years. Double-blind, placebo-controlled studies from Europe began in the 1990s. These papers were mainly from Italy and France.

In 1990, effectiveness was well documented by Tari et al. [7] using sublingual dust mite antigens for 12–18 months. Allergic rhinitis and asthma symptoms improved in the children treated. There was a significant decrease in symptoms as well as medication use. In 1994, after 24 months of treatment, the same researchers found a decrease of specific IgE antibodies to dust mites [36].

A review article by Passalacqua and Canonica [37] in 2001 reported on 18 studies using SLIT in double-blind, placebo-controlled trials. Sixteen of these studies involving the most common allergens showed improved symptoms and decreased medication in rhinitis. Studies also showed efficacy for asthma and were done in adults and children. Safety profiles were good using the current dosing regimens [9, 21, 38–40]. No life-threatening reactions have occurred.

There are various methods using local immunotherapy. Nasal immunotherapy has shown efficacy but only shows local immunologic changes [41]. Sublingual spit was not as effective as sublingual-swallow delivery. Sublingual-swallow technique has been found to be most effective. Sublingual-swallow

Table 1. SCIT dosing guidelines

Antigen	μg/potency	Effective dose	Effective concentration	Ref. No.
Dust mite	124/10,000 AU	7–11.9 μg Der p 1	1,200 AU/ml	45, 46
Dust mite	50/10,000 AU	10 μg Der f 1	4,000 AU/ml	46
Grass	370/100,000 BAU	15 μg	8,000 BAU/ml	47
Short ragweed	325/1:10 w/v	6–24 μg Amb a 1	1:30 to 1:250 w/v	48, 49

Comparison is by a monthly maintenance dose. European baseline SCIT dosage is lower than that in the US (this may account for some of the variability and higher ratios). AU = Allergy units/ml; BAU = bioequivalent units/ml.

immunotherapy shows localized as well as systemic immunologic changes [2, 7, 11, 16, 36]. The antigen, as a liquid or tablet, is held under the tongue for 20 s to 2 min and the remainder is swallowed. Doses are given up to 3 times per day. Most methods use daily doses during buildup and often less frequent doses during maintenance. In our clinic we use daily administration.

Single antigen, relatively rapid buildup protocols have been shown to effectively treat dust mites [2, 3, 5, 7, 8]. Treatment should be continued for at least 24 months. Single antigens such as trees, grass, ragweed, or other pollens can be treated by preseasonal, high-potency regimens. This can be maintained throughout the year or decreased to a lower dose during the season [17].

Doses of single antigens are 5–200 times stronger than those used for SCIT. Efficacy and safety have been shown in a wide range of dosages. The attached tables 1–4 summarize the analyses of specific studies and compare doses, dosing schedules, and results. The optimal dosing regimen has not yet been identified. The increased cost of the antigens is typically offset by the decrease in the number of office visits needed for injections.

'Threshold' dosing is a good way to start treatment for multiple antigens [33]. Using the serial end point titration technique [42], the initial doses are based on the first positive intradermal test. For multiple antigens, the drops are given 3 times per day. Doses are increased as objective improvement is seen on follow-up skin testing. Mold allergies respond particularly well to this method.

Foods can be treated based on in vitro specific IgE level testing (such as Pharmacia Unicap) or challenge testing. Dosage depends on the severity of the food allergy. The more severe food allergies require smaller doses. Antigens are used 3 times daily until tolerance develops. Specific IgE levels are rechecked typically every 6–12 months. Doses are not increased until specific IgE levels start to decline.

Table 2. Double-blind placebo controlled sublingual studies: dust mite

Reference	Number of study patients	Disease and duration	Maintenance dose/month	Results p < 0.05	Safety	Monthly maintenance dose and dose ratio		
						Der p 1	Der f 1	SLIT/SCIT ratio
Mungan et al. [5]	5 active, 11 placebo	rhinitis and asthma: 12 months	867 IR	↓ssx ↓ Med scr NC IgE D1 ↑ IgG4 12 months	1 patient buccal pruritis	N/A	N/A	86
Tari et al. [36]	30 active, 28 placebo children	rhinitis and asthma: 24 months	4,875 STU	↑ IgE D1 ↑ IgG4 18 months ↑ IgG 12 months	none	N/A	N/A	5
Bahceciler [8]	8 active, 7 placebo children	rhinitis and asthma: 5 months	69.3 µg Der p 1 121.2 µg Der f 1	↓ asthma ssx, score ↓ meds ↑ ID test ↑ peak flow	none	69.3 µg[a]	121.2 µg[a]	5.8–9.9 Der p 1[a] 12.2 Der f 1[a]
Pajno et al. [3]	12 active, 12 placebo children	asthma: 24 months	10.4 µg Der p 1 5.2 µg Der f 1	↓ meds by year 2 ↓ asthma flares ↓ noc ssx	4 fatigue, 1 lip swelling, 1 oral pruritis, no rx needed	10.4 µg[a]	5.2 µg[a]	3.25
Tari et al. [7]	30 active, 28 placebo	rhinitis and asthma: 18 months	4,875 STU	↑ ID ↓ ssx ↓ meds ↑ spec IgG	3 hives, 8 mild asthma, 4 GI	N/A	N/A	5
Guez et al. [4]	36 active, 36 placebo	rhinitis: 24 months	187 µg Der p 1 144.2 µg Der f 1	NS	2 oral pruritis	187 µg[a]	144.2 µg[a]	15.6–28.7 Der p 1[a] 14.4 Der f 1[a]
Bousquet et al. [2]	42 active, 43 placebo	rhinitis and asthma: 24 months	309.6 µg Der p 1 541.8 µg Der f 1	↓ ssx ↑ AM peak flow ↑ IgG4	3 urticaria and throat itching, 1 asthma	309.6 µg[a]	541.8 µg[a]	200
Allergy Associates of La Crosse (this study)			36 µg Der f 1				36 µg[a]	2.5–10 Der f 1[a]

European baseline SCIT dosage is lower than the US (this may account for some of the variability and higher ratios). SLIT/SCIT ratio = Sublingual immunotherapy monthly maintenance dose/subcutaneous monthly maintenance dose; IR = index of reactivity; N/A = not available; ssx = symptom scores; NC = no change; meds = medication use; ID = intradermal; NS = not significant.
[a]Calculated dosages.

Table 3. Double-blind placebo controlled sublingual studies: grass pollen

Reference	Number of study patients	Disease and duration	Maintenance dose/month	Results p < 0.05	Safety	Monthly maintenance dose and dose ratio		
						types of grass	monthly maintenance dose	SLIT/SCIT ratio
Marcucci et al. [50]	30 active, 20 control children	Seasonal allergic rhinitis: 7 months	7.5 μg	none (safety study)	no side effects or rxns	5 major grass allergens	7.5 μg[a]	0.5[a]
Di Rienzo et al. [17]	48 children 5–12 years; four groups: Pre-co, Pre-co, co, control	rhino-conjunctivitis: 5½ months	group A: 9.1 μg group B: 9.1 μg group C: 6.5 μg	↓ ssx in 3 active groups	mild edema, erythema of eyelids in 2 patients	5 grasses: Phleum, Lolium, Dactylis, Poa, Festuca	group A: 9.1 μg[a] group B: 9.1 μg[a] group C: 6.5 μg[a]	0.61[a] 0.61[a] 0.43[a]
Hordijk et al. [18]	27 active, 30 placebo	rhinitis conjunctivitis: 10 months	82,327 BU	↓ ssx	minor local symptoms	timothy, velvet, orchard, Bermuda, sweet vernal	N/A	N/A
Clavel et al. [19]	62 active, 58 placebo	rhinitis conjunctivitis: 6 months	576 μg Phl p 5	↓ ssx	oral itching; wheezing in some patients	5 major grass pollens	576 μg[a] Phl P 5	38.4[a]
Gozalo et al. [51]	35 active, 19 control (1st year: 42 active)	ocular nasal respiratory: 7 months 1st year 12 months 2nd year	81.24 BU	↓ ssx	2.7% mild rxns; some needing antihistamines	Lolium perenne (rye grass)	N/A	N/A
Quirino et al. [52]	10 active, 10 placebo	seasonal rhinitis: 12 months sublingual and injection groups	SLIT = 81.2 BU SCIT = 34.3 BU	↓ ssx meds	none reported	5 grasses: Dg, Fp, Lp, Php, Pp	N/A	2.37[a]

Table 3 (continued)

Reference	Number of study patients	Disease and duration	Maintenance dose/month	Results $p < 0.05$	Safety	Monthly maintenance dose and dose ratio		
						types of grass	Monthly maintenance dose	SLIT/SCIT ratio
Feliziani et al. [21]	18 active, 16 placebo	ocular rhinitis: 3.5–4 months	260 BU	overall ssx	none reported	orchard meadow, rye, timothy, sweet vernal	N/A	N/A
Pradalier et al. [15]	62 active, 61 placebo	ocular, rhinitis, asthma: 4.5 months	255 µg Phl P 5	ocular ssx, asthma ssx	'minor side effects'	orchard, meadow, ryegrass, sweet vernal and timothy	255 µg[a] Phl P 5	17[a]
Allergy Associates of La Crosse (this study)			270 µg			Bermuda, Kentucky blue, meadow fescue, orchard, rye, redtop, timothy sweet vernal	270 µg[a]	18[a]

European baseline SCIT dosage is lower than the US (this may account for some of the variability and higher ratios). SLIT/SCIT ratio = Sublingual immunotherapy monthly maintenance dose/subcutaneous monthly maintenance dose; N/A = not available; ssx = symptom scores; meds = medication use.
[a] Calculated dosages.

Table 4. Controlled sublingual studies: ragweed pollen

Reference	Number of study patients	Disease and duration	Maintenance dose/month	Results p < 0.05	Safety	Monthly maintenance dose and dose ratio	
						Amb a 1	SLIT/SCIT ratio
Valle et al. [53]	19 active, 14 control (meds only)	rhinitis and asthma: 3 months	36 µg Amb a 1	Nasal challenge, skin reactivity ssx	1 lip itching	36 µg	6[a]
Allergy Associates of La Crosse (this study)			180 µg Amb a 1			180 µg[a]	7–30[a]

European baseline SCIT dosage is lower than the US (this may account for some of the variability and higher ratios). SLIT/SCIT ratio = Sublingual immunotherapy monthly maintenance dose/subcutaneous monthly maintenance dose; ssx = symptom scores; meds = medication use.
[a]Calculated dosages.

Contact sensitivity to nickel can be improved using sublingual doses of nickel sulfate [43, 44]. Nickel sulfate is used to test intradermally and a sublingual dose is chosen to start that is weaker than the first positive skin reaction (using a modified serial end point titration technique) [42].

The World Health Organization position paper [31] published in 1998 found that properly conducted double-blind, placebo-controlled trials have shown the effectiveness of sublingual-swallow immunotherapy with grass, *Parietaria* and mite vaccines. The ARIA (Allergic Rhinitis and Impact on Asthma) [32] guidelines published in 2001 gave specific indications for usage.

Because of improved convenience, compliance, and safety, SLIT opens the door for expansion of immunotherapy to a first-line treatment option in allergic disease.

References

1   Donahue JG, Greineder DK, Connor-Lacke L, Canning CF, Platt R: Utilization and cost of immunotherapy for allergic asthma and rhinitis. Ann Allergy Asthma Immunol 1999;82: 339–347.

2   Bousquet J, Scheinmann P, Guinnepain MT, Perrin-Fayolle M, Sauvaget J, Tonnel AB, Pauli G, Caillaud D, Dubost R, Leynadier F, Vervloet D, Herman D, Galvain S, Andre C: Sublingual-swallow immunotherapy (SLIT) in patients with asthma due to house-dust mites: A double blind placebo-controlled study. Allergy 1999;54/3:249–260.

3   Pajno GB, Morabito L, Traina G, Bragho S, Saturno M, Barberio G, Puccinelli P: Clinical and immunological effects of long-term sublingual immunotherapy in asthmatic children sensitized to mites: A double-blind placebo controlled study. Allergy 2000;55:842–849.

4   Guez S, Vatrinet C, Fadel R, Andre C: House dust mite SLIT in perennial rhinitis: A double blind placebo controlled study. Allergy 2000;55:369–375.

5   Mungan D, Misirligil Z, Gurbuz L, et al: Comparison of the efficacy of subcutaneous and sublingual immunotherapy in mite-sensitive patients with rhinitis and asthma – A placebo controlled study. Ann Allergy Asthma Immunol 1999;82:485–490.

6   Giovane AL, Bardare M, Passalacqua G, Ruffoni S, Scordamaglia A, Ghezzi E, Canonica GW: A three-year double-blind placebo-controlled study with specific oral immunotherapy to *Dermatophagoides*: Evidence of safety and efficacy in paediatric patients. Clin Exp Allergy 1994; 24:53–59.

7   Tari MG, Mancino M, Monti G: Efficacy of sublingual immunotherapy in patients with rhinitis and asthma due to house dust mite – A double blind study. Allergol Immunopathol 1990;18/5: 277–284.

8   Bahceciler NN, Isik U, Bartan IB, Basaran MM: Efficacy of sublingual immunotherapy in children with asthma and rhinitis: A double blind, placebo-controlled study. Pediatr Pulmonol 2001;32:49–55.

9   Ariano R, Panzani RC, Augeri G: Efficacy and safety of oral immunotherapy in respiratory allergy to *Parietaria judaica* pollen: A double-blind study. J Invest Allergol Clin Immunol 1998;8/3: 155–160.

10 Troise C, Voltolini S, Canessa A, Pecora S, Negrini AC: Sublingual immunotherapy in *Parietaria* pollen-induced rhinitis: A double-blind study. J Invest Allergol Clin Immunol 1995;5/1:25–30.

11 Passalacqua G, Albano M, Riccio A, Fregonese L, Puccinelli P, Parmiani S, Canonica GW: Clinical and immunologic effects of a rush sublingual immunotherapy to *Parietaria* species: A double-blind, placebo-controlled trial. J Allergy Clin Immunol 1999;104:964–968.

12 La Rosa M, Ranno C, Andre C, Carat F, Tosca MA, Canonica GW: Double-blind placebo-controlled evaluation of sublingual-swallow immunotherapy with standardized *Parietaria judaica* extract in children with allergic rhinoconjunctivitis. J Allergy Clin Immunol 1999;104:425–432.

13 Purello DA, Gangemi S, Isola S, La Motta N, Puccinelli P, Parmiani S, Savi E, Ricciardi L: Sublingual immunotherapy: A double-blind placebo-controlled trial with *Parietaria judaica* extract standardized in mass units in patients with rhinoconjunctivitis asthma or both. Allergy 1999;54:968–973.

14 Clavel R, Andre C, Bousquet J: Reduction of corticosteroid therapy by sublingual immunotherapy. Double blind study against placebo of standardised 5 grass pollen extract in rhinitis. Allergy 1995;50/26:279.

15 Pradalier A, Basset D, Claudel A, Couturier P, Wessel F, Galvain S, Andre C: Sublingual-swallow immunotherapy (SLIT) with a standardized five-grass-pollen extract (drops and sublingual tablets) versus placebo in seasonal rhinitis. Allergy 1999;54:819–828.

16 Fanta C, Bohle B, Hirt W, Siemann U, Horak F, Kraft D, Ebner H, Ebner C: Systemic immunological changes induced by administration of grass pollen allergens via the oral mucosa during sublingual immunotherapy. Int Arch Allergy Immunol 1999;120:218–224.

17 Di Rienzo V, Puccinelli P, Frati F, Parmiani S: Grass pollen specific sublingual/swallow immunotherapy in children: Open-controlled comparison among different treatment protocols. Allergol Immunopathol 1999;27/3:145–151.

18 Hordijk GJ, Antvelink JB, Luwema RA: Sublingual immunotherapy with a standardised grass pollen extract; a double-blind placebo-controlled study. Allergol Immunopathol 1998;26/5:234–240.

19 Clavel R, Bousquet J, Andre C: Clinical efficacy of sublingual-swallow immunotherapy: A double-blind, placebo-controlled trial of standardized five-grass-pollen extract in rhinitis. Allergy 1998;53:493–498.

20 Sabbah A, Hassoun S, Le Sellin J, Andre C, Sicard H: A double-blind, placebo-controlled trial by the sublingual route of immunotherapy with a standardized grass pollen extract. Allergy 1994;49:309–313.

21 Feliziani V, Lattuada G, Parmiani S, Dall'Aglio PP: Safety and efficacy of sublingual rush immunotherapy with grass allergen extracts: A double-blind study. Allergol Immunopathol 1995;23/5:224–230.

22 Van Deusen MA, Angelini B, Cordoro KM, Seiler BA, Wood L, Skoner DP: Efficacy and safety of oral immunotherapy with short ragweed extract. Ann Allergy Asthma Immunol 1997;78:573–580.

23 Vourdas D, Syrigou E, Potamianou P, Carat F, Batard T, Andre C, Papageorgiou PS: Double-blind, placebo-controlled evaluation of sublingual immunotherapy with standardized olive pollen extract in pediatric patients with allergic rhinoconjunctivitis and mild asthma due to olive pollen sensitization. Allergy 1998;53:662–672.

24 Horak F: Immunotherapy with sublingual birch pollen extract. A short-term double blind placebo study. J Investig Allergol Clin Immunol 1998;8/3:165–171.

25 Nucera E, Schiavino D, D'Ambrosio C, Stabile A, Rumi C, Gasbarrini G, Patriarca G: Immunological aspects of oral desensitization in food allergy. Dig Dis Sci 2000;45:637–641.

26 Patriarca G, Schiavino D, Nucera E, Schinco G, Milani A, Gasbarrini GB, et al: Food allergy in children: Results of a standardized protocol for oral desensitization. Hepatogastroenterology 1998;45/19:52–58.

27 Mastrandrea F, Serio G, Minelli M, Minardi A, Scarcia G, Coradduzza G, Parmiani S: Specific sublingual immunotherapy in atopic dermatitis: Results of a 6-year follow-up of 35 consecutive patients. Allergol Immunopathol 2000;28/2:54–62.

28 Bagnasco M: Absorption and distribution kinetics of the major *Parietaria* allergen administered by noninjectable routes to healthy human beings. J Allergy Clin Immunol 1997;100:13–18.

29 Bagnasco M, Passalacqua G, Villa G, Augeri C, Flamigni G, Borini E, Falagiani P, Mistrello G, Canonica GW, Mariani G: Pharmacokinetics of an allergen and a monomeric allergoid for oromucosal immunotherapy in allergic volunteers. Clin Exp Allergy 2001;31:54–60.

30 Brown JL, Frew AJ: The efficacy of oromucosal immunotherapy in respiratory allergy. Clin Exp Allergy 2001;31/1:8–10.

31   Bousquet J, Lockey R, Malling HJ: Allergen immunotherapy: Therapeutic vaccines for allergic diseases. World Health Organization Position Paper. Allergy 1998;53(suppl 44)1–29.

32   Bousquet J: ARIA Workshop Group Guidelines. J Allergy Clin Immunol 2001;108:S242–S245.

33   Morris DL: Current use of sublingual-swallow immunotherapy. Curr Opin Otolaryngol Head Neck Surg 2001;9/3:179–180.

34   Morris DL: Use of sublingual antigen in diagnosis and treatment of food allergy. Ann Allergy 1969;27:289–294.

35   Morris DL: Treatment of respiratory disease with ultra-small doses of antigens. Ann Allergy 1970;28:494–500.

36   Tari MG, Mancino M, Madonna F, Buzzoni L, Parmiani S: Immunologic evaluation of 24 month course of sublingual immunotherapy. Allergol Immunopathol 1994;22/5:209–216.

37   Passalacqua G, Canonica GW: Allergen-specific sublingual immunotherapy for respiratory allergy. BioDrugs 2001;15:509–519.

38   Lombardi C: Safety of sublingual immunotherapy with monomeric allergoid in adults: Multicenter post-marketing surveillance study. Allergy 2001;56:989–992.

39   Andre C: Safety of sublingual immunotherapy in children and adults. Int Arch Allergy Immunol 2000;121:229–234

40   Di Rienzo V: Post-marketing surveillance study on the safety of sublingual immunotherapy in children. Allergy 1999;54:1110–1113.

41   Giannarini L, Maggi E: Decrease of allergen-specific T cell response induced by local nasal immunotherapy. Clin Exp Allergy 1998;28:547–551.

42   Nadarajah R, Rechtweg JS, Corey JP: Introduction to serial endpoint titration. Immunol Allergy Clin North Am 2001;21:369–381.

43   Panzani RC, Schiavino D, Nucera E, Pellegrino S, Fais G, Schinco G, Patriarca G: Oral hyposensitization to nickel allergy: Preliminary clinical results. Int Arch Allergy Immunol 1995;107/1–3: 251–254.

44   Morris DL: Intradermal testing and sublingual desensitization for nickel. Cutis 1998;6/3:129–132.

45   Ewan P, Alexander M, Snape C: Effective hyposensitization in allergic rhinitis using a potent partially purified extract of house dust mite. Clin Allergy 1988;18:501–508.

46   Olsen O, Larsen K, Jacobsan L, Svendsen U: A 1-year, placebo-controlled, double-blind house-dust-mite immunotherapy study in asthmatic adults. Allergy 1997;52:853–859.

47   Dolz I, Martinez-Cocera C, Bartolome J: A double-blind, placebo-controlled study of immunotherapy with grass-pollen extract Alutard SQ during a 3-year period with initial rush immunotherapy. Allergy 1996;51:489–500.

48   Creticos P, Adkinson N, Kagey-Sobotka A: Nasal challenge with ragweed pollen in hayfever patients: Effect of immunotherapy. J Clin Invest 1985;76:2247–2253.

49   Furin M, Norman P, Creticos P: Immunotherapy decreases antigen-induced eosinophil cell migration into the nasal cavity. J Allergy Clin Immunol 1991;88:27–32.

50   Marcucci F, Sensi L, Frati F, Senna GE, Canonica GW, Parmiani S, Passalacqua G: Sublingual tryptase and ECP in children treated with grass pollen sublingual immunotherapy (SLIT): Safety and immunologic implications. Allergy 2001;56:1091–1095.

51   Gozalo F, Martin S, Rico P, Alvarez E, Cortes C: Clinical efficacy and tolerance of two year *Lolium perenne* sublingual immunotherapy. Allergol Immunopathol 1997;25/5:219–227.

52   Quirino T, Iemoli E, Siciliani S, Parmiani S, Milazzo F: Sublingual versus injective immunotherapy in grass pollen allergic patients: A double blind (double dummy) study. Clin Exp Allergy 1996;26:1253–1261.

53   Valle C, Bazzi S, Berra D, Sillano V, Puccinelli P, Parmiani S: Effects of sublingual immunotherapy in patients sensitised to *Ambrosia*. An open controlled study. Allergol Immunopathol 2000; 28:311–317.

David L. Morris, MD
Allergy Associates of La Crosse Ltd.,
615 South 10th Street, La Crosse, WI 54602–2408 (USA)
Tel. +1 608 782 2027, Fax +1 608 782 6172, E-Mail dmorris@allergysolutions.com

Markert UR, Elsner P (eds): Local Immunotherapy in Allergy.
Chem Immunol Allergy. Basel, Karger, 2003, vol 82, pp 11–24

....

Mucosal Immunity – Mucosal Tolerance

A Strategy for Treatment of Allergic Diseases

Ursula Wiedermann

Department of Pathophysiology, University of Vienna,
Vienna, Austria

Key Words

MALT · Mucosal vaccination · Mucosal tolerance · Nasal/oral inhalation · Treatment agent allergies · Hyperresponsiveness

Abstract

The mucosal surfaces of the respiratory, the gastrointestinal and the urogenital tract, covering a total of $300\,m^2$, are the largest areas within the body in contact with the external environment and thus are major sites of antigen exposure. Discriminating between pathogenic antigens, towards which a protective immune response has to be established, and harmless antigens – such as food, airborne antigens or the commensal bacterial flora – that should be ignored is the most challenging task of the mucosal immune system. In order to handle these challenges the mucosal immune system has generated two arms of adaptive defenses: (1) antigen exclusion performed by secretory IgA and secretory IgM antibodies to modulate or inhibit adherence or colonization of microorganisms and prevent penetration of potentially dangerous antigens (toxins, etc.), and (2) suppressive mechanisms to avoid local and peripheral overreaction against innocuous substances contacting the mucosal surfaces. The latter arm is referred to as oral or mucosal tolerance. A breakdown or a failure of induction of long-lasting tolerance to environmental and food antigens or components of the indigenous microflora is believed to lead to allergic diseases or food enteropathies. Based on the physiological situation to prevent hypersensitivity reactions, tolerance induction via the mucosa has been proposed as a treatment strategy against human inflammatory diseases, such as allergies.

The Mucosal Immune System

Mucosal surfaces of the gut, the respiratory and urogenital tract have pleiotropic tasks that include absorption of nutrients, transport of macromolecules as well as barrier and secretory functions. As these mucosal surfaces are the largest areas within the body – mucosae span an area of $300 \, m^2$, whereas the skin surface covers only $2 \, m^2$ – they are constantly exposed to millions of potentially harmful antigens, such as environmental antigens, food or different microorganisms. Therefore, the mucosal surfaces need effective protection, which is achieved by unspecific and specific defense mechanisms. Epithelial structures, ciliated epithelium, mucus, gastric acid and antimicrobial substances (lysozyme, lactoferrin, lactoperoxidase) serve as a first line of defense. In addition, the mucosal surfaces are protected by a highly developed and specialized immune system, the mucosa-associated lymphoid system (MALT), which involves the majority (up to 80%) of immunologically active cells in the body.

The basic features of the mucosal immune system include a strongly developed innate defense system (phagocytosis, generation of anitmicrobial molecules, antigen presentation by epithelial cells) and particular populations of lymphocytes, which differ in their origin, phenotype or their secretion products from those belonging to the systemic immune system. Moreover, the migration of cells originating from the intestine or the bronchi to mucosae of organs and exocrine glands (homing of lymphocytes), the transport of polymeric immunoglobulin (sIgA, sIgM) through the epithelium into the lumen, or the induction of immunological unresponsiveness to luminal antigen (mucosal tolerance) are important characteristics of this immune system [1] (table 1).

MALT: Common Mucosal Immune System
The MALT consists of solitary and multiple lymphoid follicles within the mucosa as well as dispersed lymphocytes within and below the epithelium, i.e. the intraepithelial lymphocytes (IEL) or the lamina propria lymphocytes (LPL), respectively. The largest and most intensively studied component of the MALT is located in the gastrointestinal tract, termed GALT [2]. The GALT comprises the Peyer's patches, mesenteric lymph nodes, the appendix and numerous solitary lymphoid follicles, especially in the large bowel. Similar structures can be found in the bronchial mucosa, termed bronchus-associated lymphoid tissue (BALT) [3], where immune responses analog to those in GALT can be induced, although the antigenic stimuli are less intensive than in the gut. Induction of mucosal responses can also occur in the palatine tonsils and other lymphoepithelial structures of Waldeyer's pharyngeal ring, including the nasal-associated lymphoid tissue (NALT), such as the adenoids in humans [4].

Table 1. Major tasks being fulfilled by the mucosal immune system

Anti-infectious defense: protection from adhesion and invasion of harmful pathogens and toxins

Barrier function and immune exclusion: protection from uptake and penetration of nondegradable potentially harmful foreign antigens into the circulation

Mucosal tolerance: protection from hypersensitivity reactions towards harmless environmental and food antigens

Mucosal homeostasis: induction of immunoregulatory functions, maintenance of an intact endogenous microflora

These MALT are structurally and functionally divided into two sites – the inductive sites for antigen uptake and processing on the one hand, and the effector sites engaging lymphocytes/plasma cells, granulocytes and mast cells, on the other hand.

The inductive sites are all compact lymphoid structures in the mucosae, comprising germinal centers formed by differentiating B cells, T cells located in the interfollicular region around the venules with high endothelium, and a variety of (mature and immature) antigen-presenting cell (APC) subsets. These organized follicles are covered by a specific follicle-associated epithelium, which contains membranous epithelial cells, called M cells. These M cells adsorb antigens (especially when particulate in nature) and transfer them from the lumen into the follicles (e.g. Peyer's patches) to the dendritic cells (DC) in order to activate T and B cells and induce mucosal immunity [5].

The effector sites are represented by lymphocytes diffusely located in the epithelium (IEL) and in the lamina propria (LPL) [6]. The IEL are primarily CD8+ T cells, characterized by the CD45 RO phenotype, the integrin αEβ7, and the presence of perforin and serine esterases in cytoplasmic granules. Due to these granules the IEL have important defense properties. The LPL are the most important mucosal effector cells. These are, on the one hand, T cells, mainly CD4+, of which so-called regulatory T cells – characterized by a particular cytokine production profile – are responsible for induction of suppressive activities (see mucosal tolerance). B cells, on the other hand, are mainly represented by IgA-producing plasma cells. The secretory IgA belongs to the polymeric form of IgA in contrast to serum monomeric IgA, which is produced in the bone marrow. The advantage of the secretory IgA is that it is mostly resistant to cleavage by bacterial proteases. IgA is the major specific humoral defense factor on mucosal surfaces and external secretions, which blocks the adhesion of bacteria to mucosal surfaces, neutralizes viral and toxic antigens and prevents the penetration of antigen into the internal environment of the organism [7].

Homing of Immunocompetent Cells

Immune responses induced by immunization via the mucosal (nasal, oral, rectal, vaginal) route are not only elicited at the site of immunization, but also occur at remote mucosal surfaces and exocrine glands. This occurs when lymphocytes, after they have contacted specific antigen within the lymphoid tissue, migrate through the lymph route and then through the blood and finally return and colonize mucosal surfaces and exocrine glands. There they develop to mature effector cells, e.g. IgA-producing plasma cells. This migration process is called 'homing', which is achieved by specific adhesion molecules – $\alpha4\beta7$ integrin – on the surface of lymphocytes which bind to the mucosal vessel adhesin MdCAM-1 on endothelial cells of mucosal capillaries [8, 9]. One example for this homing process, which is the key function of the 'common mucosal immune system', is the migration of cells originating from the intestine to the mammary glands, resulting in the presence of sIgA and cells with specificities against intestinal antigens (enteromammary axis) [10].

Nevertheless, there is also accumulating evidence that a certain regionalization exists in the mucosal immune system, in particular a dichotomy between the gut and the upper respiratory tract. Differences in the antigenic repertoire, adhesion molecules or chemokines involved in leukocyte extravasation might explain this disparity. Primed immune cells may tend to home to the effector sites corresponding to the inductive sites, where the initial antigen contact took place. Such regionalization within the common mucosal immune system has to be taken into account in the development of certain mucosal vaccines [11].

Mucosal Tolerance

Immunological tolerance is a fundamental property of the immune system allowing for the discrimination between self and non-self antigens. Self-tolerance may be induced in generative lymphoid organs (i.e. thymus, bone marrow) as a consequence of immature self-reactive lymphocytes recognizing self-antigen, called central tolerance [12]. However, since not all self-reactive lymphocytes are eliminated in the primary lymphoid organs – either because certain self-antigens are not expressed in the thymus or due to escaping from the selection processes – the immune system must regulate the potentially self-reactive lymphocytes in the periphery. This process is called peripheral tolerance [13]. A failure in maintaining unresponsiveness to self-antigens can result in the development of autoimmunity.

The same mechanisms of peripheral unresponsiveness exist also against foreign – mainly soluble – antigens, in order to prevent the organisms from untoward immunological immune responses against innocuous substances. Peripheral tolerance induction to foreign antigen can be induced by systemic antigen application or by mucosal administration of antigen called mucosal tolerance.

Mucosal tolerance is a meanwhile well-accepted phenomenon, which was initially referred to as 'oral tolerance', because it was first recognized after feeding antigen [14]. As immunological unresponsiveness – characterized by a refractory or diminished capability to develop an immune response upon systemic reexposure to the specific antigen – can also be achieved after antigen administration via the nasal, inhalative, rectal or genital route, it is now more broadly referred to as mucosal tolerance.

Mucosal tolerance is believed to be an important physiological mechanism, whereby the continued high-load exposure to harmless environmental airborne and food antigens or to products of the commensal microflora is tolerated and the development of hypersensitivity reactions to these antigens is inhibited. A breakdown or a failure in maintaining tolerance towards these antigens is therefore thought to be causally related to the development of allergic diseases and food enteropathies [15, 16].

Experimental Models of Mucosal Tolerance

An anecdotal report that oral ingestion of antigen might modify subsequent systemic immune responses was first found in 1826 by Dakin [17], describing that South American Indians ate poison ivy leaves to prevent contact sensitivity reactions to this plant. The first experimental model was established in 1911 by Wells and Osborne [18] showing that the feeding of egg protein prior to systemic challenge with the same antigen prevented the development of anaphylaxis.

Following several studies in animals it was proposed that oral tolerance induction modifies primarily Th1-biased immune responses. In experimental models of Th1-mediated autoimmune diseases, such as experimental encephalomyelitis [19], nonobese diabetes [20], myasthenia gravis [21], or experimental autoimmune uveitis [22], it was shown that oral antigen application inhibited or delayed the onset or reduced the course of the respective disease. Apart from these studies it was also demonstrated that mucosal tolerance – particularly when induced via the respiratory route – can also modify Th2-based immune responses. Holt and colleagues [23, 24] were the first demonstrating that the inhalation of the antigen ovalbumin was followed by a suppression of antigen-specific IgE and IL-4 production Other studies, using typical inhalative allergens, further demonstrated the efficacy of inhalative, intranasal or tracheal antigen administration in modulating antigen-specific immune responses, but even more also prevented pathophysiological events, such as airway inflammation or bronchial hyperreactivity [25–29]. Also models of food allergy exist that demonstrate the efficacy of oral/mucosal administration of food allergens, such as peanut allergens, to prevent or reduce intestinal inflammation and hypersecretion [30, 31].

Mechanisms of Mucosal Tolerance

It has become clear that mucosal tolerance is a very complex process that is mediated by more than one mechanism, involving suppression of some immune responses and induction of others. Several factors, such as the nature and structure of the antigen, the antigen dose, antigen presentation, components of the innate immune system, the maturation state of the immune system, the genetic background or the indigenous flora influence the immunological outcome following mucosal antigen administration. It is generally believed that unresponsiveness can be more easily achieved in T cells than in B cells. Nevertheless, the effector functions of B cells – i.e. antibody production – can be influenced by the lack of the respective T cell help. In this respect, the three major responsible mechanisms behind tolerance induction have been described to be due to clonal deletion, clonal anergy of antigen-specific T cells, or the induction of active suppression or immunodeviation, mediated by so-called regulatory T cells [32–34].

Structure/Nature of the Antigen, Antigen Dose and Frequency of
Antigen Application

Particulate antigens and pathogens (i.e. microorganisms) promote active immunity, partially because they are taken up by the M cells in the epithelium of the lymphoid follicles, e.g. Peyer's patches. Conversely, soluble antigens, towards which tolerance can be induced, may not primarily use this route, but are rather taken up by intestinal epithelial cells that might present antigen to T cells lying directly next to them in the epithelium or by APCs beneath the epithelium, which are distinct in phenotype and function from those taking up particulate/pathogenic antigens [35, 36]. Among the soluble antigens there seems to be a difference between those acting as strong tolerogens and those which are effective immunogens – the immunogenicity and tolerogenicity of an antigen may thus stand in a reciprocal relationship [37].

In the induction phase of tolerance the antigen dose and the frequency of antigen application seem to play important roles. It has been described that single high-dose antigen application (>0.5 mg/g body weight in mice) favors the induction of anergy or deletion of antigen-specific T cells [38–40], whereas multiple low dose antigen applications (<0.1 mg/g body weight in mice) are more likely to generate regulatory T cells [41]. It should be noted though that very low doses (<0.005 mg/g body weight) – at least when given orally – can prime the organism for subsequent systemic and local immune responses [42].

In terms of regulatory T cells several subtypes with a distinct cytokine secretion pattern of TGF-β, IL-10 and/or IL-4/IL-5 have been described. These T cells, expressing certain surface markers, such as CD4+CD25+, CD38+, CD45RblowCD4+(CD25–), are termed Tr, Th3 or Tr1 T cells, of which it is at the moment unclear whether they all belong to an identical T cell subpopulation and/or are derived from the same precursor T cells [43–45]. Apart from the CD4+ T cells also CD8+ T cells, inducible after inhalative or oral antigen administration, have been described to play a role in tolerance induction, mainly by mechanisms of immunodeviation [24, 46].

Role of the APCs

Antigen presentation plays an important role in the induction of mucosal tolerance. There is strong evidence that antigen can be presented to T cells by so-called nonprofessional APC, such as the intestinal epithelial cells. These cells can acquire and transport macromolecules from the lumen, they can express MHC class I and MHC class II molecules on their basolateral surface, but they do not usually express costimulatory molecules. Therefore, it has been speculated that antigen presentation by these cells would result in a tolerance of the respective T cells. Alternatively, these cells could cooperate in antigen presentation as they might give signals to professional APCs and T cells whether an antigen is dangerous or not [47, 48].

There is increasing evidence for the importance of DCs as professional APCs in the tolerance induction process [49]. It seems that particular immature DCs with a low expression of the costimulatory molecules CD80 and CD86 mediate tolerance, whereas mature DCs are important for the induction of active immunity against microorganisms [50]. In the Peyer's patches three distinct phenotypes of DCs have been described: the lymphoid CD11c+8α+ (DC1), the myeloid CD11c+11b+ (DC2), and double-negative CD11b–8α–, which can develop to either of the other phenotypes. Soluble antigens are taken up by the myeloid (CD11b+) DC2 and lead via production of TGF-β and/or IL-10 by Th3 cells to suppressive immune responses. Stimulation by microbial antigens or induction of inflammatory signals lead to the production of IL-12 by lymphoid DC1 or double-negative DCs, whereby Th1-like immune responses are initiated [36, 51]. Recently, it has been described that distinct subsets of DCs were located in the gastrointestinal and respiratory tract: DCs of the gastrointestinal tract seem to promote the development of Th3 cells by the production of TGF-β [52], whereas DCs via a preferential production of IL-10 activate Tr1 cells in the respiratory tract [53]. As previously mentioned, such cellular differences together with (or due to) different antigenic loads might be a reason for the regionalization of these two compartments within the common mucosal immune system.

Genetic Background

From experimental models it becomes apparent that certain strains of mice demonstrate a unique response pattern following immunization to an antigen (e.g. low and high IgE responder strains). However, in terms of tolerance induction it has been shown that most strains of mice can be tolerized to a large number of antigens and that there does not seem to be a clear linkage to the major histocompatibility complex haplotype or IgE responder status. Nevertheless, the degree of tolerance induction might be affected, as the antigen clearance from the circulation seems to be influenced by genetic differences [54].

Maturation State of the Immune System

It has been experimentally demonstrated that early oral introduction of antigen (ovalbumin) into mice leads to systemic sensitization instead of tolerance. Tolerance can usually be induced after 7–10 days of age, before weaning takes place at 21 days. Feeding antigen close to the day of weaning leads to a temporary reduction in the ease of tolerance induction [55]. How long this immunological window for tolerance induction actually lasts in humans is not yet known, but the general recommendation for introduction of foreign food antigens is 6 months of age.

Role of the Indigenous Flora

The presence of a normal indigenous flora plays an important role in anti-infectious resistance by competitive interaction with pathogenic bacteria, but is also important for directly influencing immune responses. This has been demonstrated in animals reared under sterile conditions (germ-free animals), showing that systemic and local immune responses are more difficult to establish and in particular that the induction of oral tolerance is unstable and short-lived [56]. Based on these findings an imbalance of the composition of the indigenous microflora is believed to play a role in the development of inflammatory diseases, such as intestinal bowel disease [16] and allergies. Indeed, differences in the intestinal colonization pattern between children of 'western lifestyle countries' with a high prevalence of allergies and of economically underdeveloped countries where allergies are less common have recently been reported [57]. Thus, intestinal colonization with a limited range of microbes due to living conditions with a high level of hygiene, termed 'hygiene theory', has become an essential factor explaining the constant increase in the prevalence of allergic diseases within the last decades [58].

Mucosal Tolerance for Treatment of Type I Allergy

In many experimental studies ovalbumin has been used as model antigen to study oral tolerance induction and the mechanisms behind this event. In particular the availability of ovalbumin-transgenic mice has proved to be of great advantage in studies on the inductive sites of immunosuppression [59]. However, with respect to experimental models of type I allergy/allergic asthma, sensitization and treatment with an inhalant rather than a dietary allergen may be closer to the situation in humans. Moreover, it is well recognized that different antigens can vary in their immunogenicity as well as their capacity to act as a tolerogen [37]. It, therefore, seems of importance to individually test the efficacy of an allergen to act as a potential therapeutic agent in a suitable model of type I allergy.

In a mouse model of aerosol sensitization to birch pollen we previously demonstrated that intranasal as well as oral administration of the major birch pollen allergen Bet v 1 prevented allergic sensitization, airway inflammation and airway hyperresponsiveness [28]. Similar effects were achieved using hypoallergenic derivates of Bet v 1, containing the immunodominant T cell peptides but not the anaphylactogenic B cell epitopes, for intranasal tolerance induction [60].

In line with other experimental studies – using the immunodominant peptides of the house dust mite allergen Der p 1 [61] or Der p 2 [62], or a major bee venom allergen [63] – we demonstrated that the prophylactic treatment with allergens via the mucosal route can induce a very potent and long-lasting immunological unresponsiveness to the respective allergen.

It has been recognized that tolerance induction in the sensitized organism is much more difficult to achieve. Crucial factors for successful therapy seem to be the exact dose, and the time and frequency of antigen application. In our model of birch pollen allergy 5 times higher doses applied in closer intervals were necessary to suppress the established allergic response [64]. The fact that tolerance in the therapeutic setup was also long-lasting (at least up to half a year) and could be induced independently of the time interval between sensitization and onset of the treatment suggested that mucosal administration of recombinant allergen could present an alternative treatment to conventional specific immunotherapy [65, 66].

Based on the fact that many allergic patients are sensitized to several unrelated allergens, tolerance induction with a panel of simultaneously applied allergens is a desirable goal. We have established a model of polysensitization to major allergens of birch and grass pollen. Intranasal tolerance with a mixture of the immunodominant peptides of the three allergens led to a marked decrease of humoral and cellular Th2-like immune responses [67]. Production of hybrid peptides or chimeric molecules, containing the immunodominant sequences of several allergens, may even enhance the efficacy of tolerance induction in polysensitized organisms, and may represent a novel form of a 'mucosal polyvalent allergy vaccine'.

As previously mentioned, the composition of the indigenous microflora seems to have an important influence on the development of allergic diseases. On the basis of recent epidemiological and clinical studies, a possible role of certain lactic acid bacteria (LAB) in the prevention of allergic diseases has become evident [68]. Experimental studies have shown a reduction of IgG1 or IgE when certain LAB were injected or orally applied with the particular allergen [69, 70].

In our mouse model of birch pollen allergy we demonstrated that intranasal and/or oral coapplication of certain LAB bacteria with the recombinant birch pollen allergen Bet v 1, prior and after sensitization with the allergen, resulted in a shift from Th2 to Th1 responses. According to a recent study using recombinant LAB expressing the house dust mite allergen Der p 1 [71], we recently evaluated the efficacy of such a mucosal allergen-delivery system not only in modulating but also significantly suppressing the allergic immune responses [72] (table 2).

Concluding Remarks

From the variety of experimental studies it becomes obvious that mucosal administration is a powerful tool for modulating immune responses. Apart from the importance to test the effectiveness and the mechanisms of action of any allergen of interest as a potential antiallergic agent or tolerogen in animal models, prophylactic treatment strategies could be of interest in patients with a known risk to develop allergy.

It is of particular clinical relevance to test the effects of mucosal allergen application in already sensitized organisms. The obvious advantage of the use of so-called hypoallergenic molecules lies in their risk-free application. Thus, the practical consequences from such experimental studies could include the development of low-risk mucosal vaccines based on the induction of tolerance – with or without the use of certain mucosal antigen delivery systems.

In comparison to conventional immunotherapy, the use of mucosal vaccines could have tremendous advantages, such as the ease of application leading to a better compliance of the patient and/or the application of patient-tailored constructs with increased efficacy and reduced anaphylactic side reactions.

Table 2. Examples of experimental models using mucosal tolerance as treatment strategy

	Immunization antigen	Mucosally applied antigen	Effects/target organs
Autoimmune disease			
EAE	MBP peptide 71–90	MBP peptide 21–40	Brain [19]
Diabetes	NOD mice	Insulin, GAD	Pancreatic island [20]
Myasthenia gravis	AChR	AChR	Prevention of muscle weakness [21]
Uveitis	S-Ag, IRBP	S-Ab	Prevention of uveitis [22]
Type I allergy			
Birch pollen	Bet v 1/BP aerosol	Bet v 1 prior to sensitization	Reduction of IgE, IgG1, IgG2a IL-4, IL-5, IFN-γ eosinophilia, AHR [28]
Birch pollen	Bet v 1/BP aerosol	Bet v 1 after sensitization	Reduction of IgE, IL-4, IL-5, eosinophilia [66]
House dust mite	Der p 1	Der p 1 peptide	Reduction of DTH, IL-2, IFN-γ, IL-4 [25]
House dust mite	Der f 2	Der f 2 (C8/119S) mutant	Down regulation of CD23 expression on B cells [62]
Bee venom	PLA$_2$	PLA$_2$ peptides	Reduction of IgE, IL-4; increase of IgG2a, IFN-γ [63]

MBP = Myelin basic protein; NOD mice = nonobese diabetic mice; GAD = glutamic acid decarboxylase; AChR = acetylcholine receptor; S-Ag, IRBP = S-antigen and interphotoreceptor retinoid binding protein; Bet v 1 = major birch pollen allergen; BP = birch pollen; Der p 1 = major house dust mite allergen (*Dermatophagoides pteronyssinus*); Der f 2 = major house dust mite allergen (*Dermatophagoides farinae*); PLA$_2$ = phospholipase A$_2$ from bee venom.

References

1   Ogra PL, Mesteky J, Lamm ME, Strober W, Bienenstock J, McGhee J: Mucosal Immunology. New York, Academic Press, 1999.
2   Brandtzaeg P: Development and basic mechanisms of human gut immunity. Nutr Rev 1998;56:S5–S18.
3   Tschernig T, Pabst R: Bronchus-associated lymphoid tissue (BALT) is not present in the normal adult lung but in different diseases. Pathobiology 2000;68:1–8.
4   Kupfer CF, Koornstra PJ, Hameleers D, Biewenga J, Spit B, Duijvestijn A, Vriesman P, Sminia T: The role of the nasopharyngeal lymphoid tissue. Immunol Today 1992;13:219–224.
5   Hathaway LJ, Kraehenbuhl JP: The role of M cells in mucosal immunity. Cell Mol Life Sci 2000;57:323–332.
6   Bailey M, Plunkett FJ, Rothkötter H-J, Vega-Lopez MA, Haverson K, Stokes CR: Regulation of mucosal immune responses in effector sites. Proc Nutr Soc 2001;60:427–435.

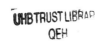

7   Mestecky J, Russel MW, Elson CO: Intestinal IgA: Novel views on its function in the defence of the large mucosal surfaces. Gut 1999;44:2–5.

8   Berlin C, Berg EL, Briskin MJ: Alpha 4 beta 7 integrin mediates lymphocytes binding to the mucosal vascular addressin MAdCAM-1. Cell 1993;74:185–195.

9   Salami L, Jalkanen S: Molecules controlling lymphocyte migration to the gut. Gut 1999;45:148–153.

10   Tlaskalova H, Vetvicka V, Lodinova R, Cerna J: Immunological components of colostrum and milk: Their origin and function. Sci Techn Froid 1982;2:133–142.

11   Brandtzaeg P, Baekkevold ES, Farstad IN: Regional specialization in the mucosal immune system: What happens in the microcompartments? Immunol Today 1999;20:141–151.

12   Ramsdell F, Lantz T, Fowlkes B: A nondeletional mechanisms of thymic self tolerance. Science 1989;246:1038–1041.

13   Rocha B, von Boehmer H: Peripheral selection of the T cell repertoire. Science 1991;251:1225–1228.

14   Brandtzaeg P: History of oral tolerance and mucosal immunity. Ann NY Acad Sci 1996;778:1–27.

15   Mowat AM: Oral tolerance and regulation of immunity to dietary antigens; in Ogra P, Mestecky J, Lamm ME, Strober W, McGhee M, Bienenstock J (eds): in Handbook of Mucosal Immunology. San Diego, Academic Press 1994, pp 185–201.

16   Duchmann R, Kaiser I, Hermann E, Mayet W, Ewe K, Buschenfelde KHM: Tolerance exists towards resident intestinal flora but is broken in active inflammatory bowel disease (IBD). Clin Exp Immunol 1995;102:448–455.

17   Dakin R: Am J Med Sci 1829;4:98–100.

18   Wells HG, Osborne TB: The biological reactions of the vegetable proteins. I. Anaphylaxis. J Infect Dis 1911;8:66–124.

19   Burkhart C, Liu GY, Anderton SM, Metzler B, Wraith DC: Peptide-induced T cell regulation of experimental autoimmune encephalomyelitis: A role for IL-10. Int Immunol 1999;11:1625–1634.

20   Maron R, Melican N, Weiner H: Regulatory Th2-type T cell lines against insulin and GAD peptides derived from orally and nasally treated NOD mice suppress diabetes. J Autoimmun 1999;12:251–258.

21   Li HL, Shi FD, Bai XF: Nasal tolerance to experimental autoimmune myasthenia gravis: Tolerance reversal by nasal administration of minute amount of IFN-γ. Clin Immunopathol 1998;87:15–22.

22   Thurau S, Wildner G: Oral tolerance for treating uveitis – New hope for an old immunological mechanism. Prog Retin Eye Res 2002;21:577–589.

23   Holt PG, Batty JE, Turner KG: Inhibition of specific IgE responses in mice by pre-exposure to inhaled antigen. Immunology 1981;42:409–417.

24   McMenamin C, Pimm C, McKersey M, Holt P: Regulation of IgE responses to inhaled antigen in mice by antigen-specific γδ T cells. Science 1994;265:1869–1871.

25   Hoyne G, Askonas BA, Hetzel C, Thomas WR, Lamb JR: Regulation of house dust mite responses by intranasally administered peptide: Transient activation of CD4+ T cell responses precedes the development of tolerance in vivo. Int Immunol 1996;7:335–342.

26   Yasue M, Yokota T, Kajiwara Y, Suko M, Okudaira H: Inhibition of airway inflammation in Der f 2 sensitized mice by oral administration of recombinant Der f 2. Cell Immunol 1997;181:30–37.

27   Lowrey J, Savage J, Palliser D, Corsin-Jimenez M, Forsyth L, Hall G, Lindey S, Stewart G, Tan K, Hoyne G, Lamb J: Induction of tolerance via the respiratory mucosa. Int Arch Allergy Immunol 1998;116:93–102.

28   Wiedermann U, Jahn-Schmid B, Bohle B, Repa A, Renz H, Kraft D, Ebner C: Suppression of antigen-specific T and B cell responses by intranasal or oral administration of recombinant Bet v 1, the major birch pollen allergen, in a murine model of type I allergy. J Allergy Clin Immunol 1999;103:1202–1210.

29   Jarnicki A, Takao T, Thomas WR: Inhibition of mucosal and systemic Th2-type immune responses by intranasal peptides containing a dominant T cell epitope of the allergen Der p 1. Int Immunol 2001;13:1223–1231.

30   Lee SY, Huang CK, Zhang TF, Schofiled BH, Burks AW, Bannon GA, Sampson HA, Li XM: Oral administration of IL-12 suppresses anaphylactic reactions in a murine model of peanut hypersensitivity. Clin Immunol 2001;101:220–228.

31 Sha U, Walker WA: Pathophysiology of intestinal food allergy. Adv Pediatr 2002;49:299–316.

32 Faria A, Weiner H: Oral tolerance: Mechanisms and therapeutic applications. Adv Immunol 1999;73:153–264.

33 Garside P, Mowat AM, Khoruts A: Oral tolerance in disease. Gut 1999;44:137–142.

34 Weiner HL: Oral tolerance, an active immunological process mediated by multiple mechanisms. J Clin Invest 2000;106:935–937.

35 Garside P, Mowat A: Oral tolerance. Semin Immunol 2001;13:177–185.

36 Iwasaki A, Kelsall B: Location of distinct Peyer's patch dendritic cell subsets and their recruitment by chemokines macrophage inflammatory protein (MIP)-3α, MIP-3β, and secondary lymphoid organ chemokines. J Exp Med 2000;191:1381–1393.

37 Wiedermann U, Jahn-Schmid B, Lindblad M, Rask C, Holmgren J, Kraft D, Ebner C: Suppressive versus stimulatory effects of allergen/cholera toxoid (CTB) conjugates depending on the nature of the allergen in a murine model of type I allergy. Int Immunol 1999;11:1717–1724.

38 Chen Y, Inobe J, Marks R, Gonnella P, Kuchroo VK, Weiner HL: Peripheral deletion of antigen-reactive T cells in oral tolerance. Nature 1995;376:177–180.

39 Marth T, Zeith Z, Ludviksson B, Strober W, Kelsall B: Murine model of oral tolerance: Induction of Fas-mediated apoptosis by blockade of interleukin-12. Ann NY Acad Sci 1998;859:290–297.

40 Taams LS, van Eden W, Wauben MH: Dose-dependent induction of distinct anergic phenotypes: Multiple levels of T cell anergy. J Immunol 1999;162:1974–1981.

41 Weiner HL: Oral tolerance: Immune mechanisms and the generation of Th3 type TGF-beta-secreting regulatory cells. Microbes Infect 2001;3:947–954.

42 Strobel S, Mowat AM: Immune responses to dietary antigens: Oral tolerance. Immunol Today 1998;19:173–181.

43 Yssel H, Groux H: Characterization of T cell subpopulations involved in the pathogenesis of asthma and allergic diseases. Int Arch Allergy Immunol 2000;121:10–18.

44 Read S, Powrie F: CD4+ regulatory T cells. Curr Opin Immunol 2001;13:644–649.

45 Battaglia M, Blazer B, Roncarolo M: The puzzling world of murine regulatory cells. Microbes Infect 2002;4:559–566.

46 Grdic D, Hornquist E, Kjerrulf M, Lycke NY: Lack of local suppression in orally tolerant CD8-deficient mice reveals a critical regulatory role of CD8+ T cells in the normal gut mucosa. J Immunol 1998;160:754–762.

47 Hershberg RM, Mayer LF: Antigen processing and presentation by intestinal epithelial cells – Polarity and complexity. Immunol Today 2000;21:123–128.

48 Brandtzaeg P: Nature and function of gastrointestinal antigen presenting cells. Allergy 2001;56:16–20.

49 Jonuleit H, Schmitt E, Steinbrink K, Enk A: Dendritic cells as tools to induce anergic versus regulatory T cells. Trends Immunol 2001;22:394–400.

50 Lutz M, Schuler G: Immature, semimature and fully mature dendritic cells: Which signals induce tolerance or immunity? Trends Immunol 2002;23:445–449.

51 Neurath M, Finotto S, Glimcher L: The role of Th1/Th2 polarization in mucosal immunity. Nat Med 2002;8:567–573.

52 Weiner HL: The mucosal milieu creates tolerogenic dendritic cells and Tr1 and Th3 regulatory cells. Nat Immunol 2001;2:671–672.

53 Akbari O, DeKruyff H, Umetsu D: Pulmonary dendritic cells producing IL-10 mediate tolerance induced by respiratory exposure to antigen. Nat Immunol 2001;2:725–731.

54 Stokes CR, Swarbrick ET, Soothill JF: Genetic differences in immune exclusion and partial tolerance to ingested antigens. Clin Exp Immunol 1983;52:678–684.

55 Strobel S: Immunity induced after a feed of antigen during early life: Oral tolerance versus sensitization. Proc Nutr Soc 2001;60:437–442.

56 Cebra J, Han-Quiang J, Sterzl J, Tlaskalova H: The role of mucosal microbiota in the development and maintenance of the mucosal immune system; in Ogra PL, Mestecky J, Lamm ME, Strober W, Bienenstock J, McGhee M (eds): Mucosal Immunology. New York, Academic Press, 1999, pp 267–280.

57 Bottcher MF, Nordin EK, Sandin A, Midvedt T, Bjorksten B: Microflora-associated characteristics in faeces from allergic and non-allergic infants. Clin Exp Allergy 2000;30:1590–1596.

58 Strachan DP: Hay fever, hygiene and household size. BMJ 1989;299:1259–1260.
59 Marth T, Ring S, Schulte D, Klesch N, Strober W, Kelsall B, Stallmach A, Zeitz M: Antigen-induced mucosal T cell activation is followed by Th1 T cell suppression in continuously fed ovalbumin TCR-transgenic mice. Eur J Immunol 2000;30:3478–3486.
60 Wiedermann U, Herz U, Baier K, Vrtala S, Neuhaus-Steinmetz U, Bohle B, Dekan G, Renz H, Ebner C, Valenta R, Kraft D: Intranasal treatment with a recombinant hypoallergenic derivative of the major birch pollen allergen Bet v 1 prevents allergic sensitization and airway inflammation in mice. Int Arch Allergy Immunol 2001;126:68–77.
61 Hall G, Houghton C, Rahbek J, Lamb J, Jarman E: Suppression of allergen reactive Th2 mediated responses and pulmonary eosinophilia by intranasal administration of an immunodominant peptide is linked to IL-10 production. Vaccine 2003;21:549–561.
62 Yasue M, Yokota T, Fukada M, Takai T, Suko M, Okudaira H, Okumura Y: Hyposensitization to allergic reaction in Der f 2-sensitized mice by intranasal administration of a mutant of rDer f 2, C8/119S. Clin Exp Immunol 1998;113:1–9.
63 Astori M, Garnier C, Kettner A, Dufour N, Corradin G, Spertini F: Inducing tolerance by intranasal administration of long peptides in naive and primed CBA/J mice. J Immunol 2000;165:3497–3505.
64 Leishman AJ, Garside P, Mowat AM: Induction of oral tolerance in the primed immune system: Influence of antigen persistence and adjuvant form. Cell Immunol 2000;202:71–78.
65 Winkler B, Baier B, Wagner S, Repa A, Scheiner O, Kraft D, Wiedermann U: Mucosal tolerance as therapy of type I allergy: Intranasal application of recombinant Bet v 1, the major birch pollen allergen, leads to the suppression of allergic immune responses and airway inflammation in sensitized mice. Clin Exp Allergy 2002;32:30–36.
66 Winkler B, Baier K, Wagner S, Repa A, Scheiner O, Kraft D, Wiedermann U: Mucosal tolerance induced in primed mice is long-lasting independent of the time of induction. Allergy 2002;57 (suppl 75):31.
67 Hufnagl K, Winkler B, Focke M, Baier K, Valenta R, Kraft D, Wiedermann U: Induction of mucosal tolerance by coapplication of recombinant Bet v 1, the major birch pollen allergen, recombinant Phl p 1 and Phl p 5, major grass pollen allergens, in polysensitized mice. Allergy 2002;57(suppl 73):49.
68 Isolauri E, Rautava S, Kalliomaki M, Kirjavainen P, Salminen S: Probiotic research: Learn from evidence. Allergy 2002;57:1076–1077.
69 Matsuzaki T, Yamazaki R, Hashimoto S, Yokokura T: The effect of oral feeding of *Lactobacillus casei* strain Shiroto on immunoglobulin E production in mice. J Dairy Sci 1998;81:48–53.
70 Shida K, Takahashi R, Iwadate E: *Lactobacillus casei* strain Shiroto suppresses serum immunoglobulin E and immunoglobulin G1 responses and systemic anaphylaxis in a food allergy model. Clin Exp Allergy 2002;32:563–570.
71 Kruisselbrink A, Heijne Den Bak-Glashouwer MJ, Havenith CE, Thole JE, Janssen R: Recombinant *Lactobacillus plantarum* inhibits house dust mite-specific T cell responses. Clin Exp Immunol 2001;126:2–8.
72 Repa A, Grangette C, Baier K, Daniel C, Kraft D, Breitender H, Mercenier A, Wiedermann U: Lactic acid bacteria – Promising tools for immunomodulation of type I allergies. Allergy 2002;57(suppl 73):72.

Ursula Wiedermann, MD, PhD
Department of Pathophysiology, Division Specific Prophylaxis and Tropical Medicine,
University of Vienna, Währinger Gürtel 18–20, A–1090 Vienna (Austria)
Tel. +43 1 40400 5132, Fax +43 1 40400 5130, E-Mail ursula.wiedermann@akh-wien.ac.at

Markert UR, Elsner P (eds): Local Immunotherapy in Allergy.
Chem Immunol Allergy. Basel, Karger, 2003, vol 82, pp 25–32

....

Antigen Resorption from the Gastrointestinal Tract

A Historical Perspective on the Pathophysiological Foundation of Modern Sublingual/Oral Immunotherapy

Wolfgang Jorde[a], Ulrich P. Jorde[b]

[a] Mönchengladbach, Germany;
[b] Columbia Presbyterian Medical Center, New York, N.Y., USA

Key Words

Allergen · Protein · Resorption · Gastrointestinal · Immunotherapy

Abstract

Resorption of small particles and proteins through the mucous membranes of the intestines has been extensively studied for well over a 100 years and the arrival of sublingual/oral immunotherapy in clinical practice has renewed interest in this process. The first line of immune response to a potential allergen is at the site of contact with a mucous membrane and both inhaled and ingested allergens usually lead to some level of direct clinically appreciable manifestation on the mucous membrane. The initial process of antigen resorption has been relatively well understood for almost one century; however, the metabolic and/or immunological fate of large particles is the subject of more recent studies. We now recognize that resorption and hematogenous spread of biologically intact allergens from the gastrointestinal tract occur despite extensive predigestion of particles and proteins within the gastrointestinal lumen and this phenomenon provides the pathophysiological underpinning of modern sublingual/oral immunotherapy.

Resorption of small particles and proteins through mucous membranes of the intestines has been extensively studied for well over a 100 years [9, 18], but it was not until the recent approval by the WHO in 1998 that sublingual/oral immunotherapy has gained general acceptance [3]. The arrival of sublingual/oral immunotherapy in clinical practice has renewed interest in the mechanisms of antigen resorption from the gastrointestinal tract. The purpose of this review is not only to illustrate the pathophysiological underpinnings of sublingual/oral immunotherapy, but equally to credit the remarkable accomplishments of clinical scientists over almost two centuries that laid the foundation for this now highly efficacious treatment modality [16].

'When talking about resorption of large molecules, one must first define large molecules. In general, large molecules have a molecular weight exceeding 10.000 kilo Dalton and may include particles and bacteria in the micrometer range. It is well known that particles of this size are digested by acid and enzymes in the gastrointestinal tract. This breakdown results in smaller molecules such as amino acids, sugars, and fats. It is less well known that large molecules can also be absorbed directly through the lymphatic system and the latter mechanism may lead to direct absorption of very large particles such as pollen, latex, seeds, and various bacteria, all of which have not undergone enzymatic predigestion' [26].

Resorption of Particles

As early as 1844 Herbst [13] described resorption of undigested large particles directly through the intestinal lymphatic system and ductus thoracicus into the bloodstream. These experiments were undertaken in dogs and later validated by Österlen (1846), Eberhard (1851), Martels (1854) and Voigt (1911) as well as Verzàrh (1928) [33].

The first line of immune response to a potential allergen is at the site of contact with a mucous membrane and both inhaled and ingested allergens usually lead to some level of direct manifestations on the respective mucous membrane. Accordingly, attempts to influence the immune response directly at the level of the mucous membrane had been made long before the exact mechanisms of the clinical manifestations (such as rash, colitis, bronchitis) were understood. Darkin [8] reported in 1829 that Native Americans successfully prevented the severe dermatitis associated with poison ivy exposure by chewing small amounts of this plant on a regular basis. This may indeed be the first clinical description of oral immunotherapy. Reports of desensitization to food allergens were published in the medical literature before the turn of the century and Curtis [7] first reported a similar success with inhaled allergens causing hay fever in 1900. Until 1930, when Fisher [10] first described resorption of yeast, a living organism, from the gastrointestinal tract of dogs, all reports had been on inert particles.

In 1960, Volkheimer [31] elegantly demonstrated resorption of starch from the human gastrointestinal tract and its appearance in blood and urine as early as 30–60 min after ingestion reaching peak concentrations after approximately 2 h.

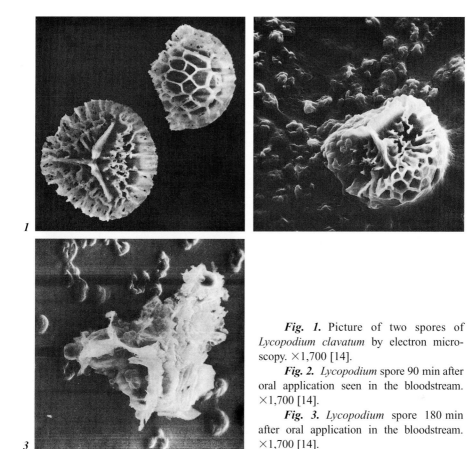

Fig. 1. Picture of two spores of *Lycopodium clavatum* by electron microscopy. ×1,700 [14].

Fig. 2. *Lycopodium* spore 90 min after oral application seen in the bloodstream. ×1,700 [14].

Fig. 3. *Lycopodium* spore 180 min after oral application in the bloodstream. ×1,700 [14].

Volkheimer further demonstrated resorption of particles as large as 65 μm (polyvinyl chloride) and initially referred to this process as 'persorption'.

The initial process of antigen resorption has thus been relatively well understood for almost a century; however, the metabolic and/or immunological fate of large particles is a topic of more recent studies and the metabolic breakdown of *Lycopodium* spores and pollen of cultivated ryegrass only a few hours following resorption was first reported in 1974 [14]. Figures 1–3 illustrate the degradation process of *Lycopodium* spores.

Resorption of Proteins

It is commonly assumed that proteins undergo enzymatic digestion in the gastrointestinal tract and thus do not enter the bloodstream as physiologically

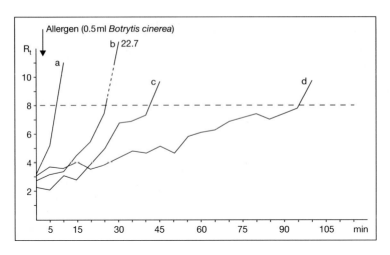

Fig. 4. Individual reactions of the bronchial system measured by body plethysmography in 4 patients given the same amount of allergen extract (0.5 ml *Botrytis cinerea*) [15].

functioning units [16]. This barrier function of the gastrointestinal tract serves to limit presentation of proteins as antigens, but Voit and Bauer [30] demonstrated as early as 1869 that this protective mechanism can be overcome by simply presenting a very large amount of substrate. It took over a 100 years to realize that his observations were not just an artificially induced oddity, but carry substantial clinical significance. Intestinal absorption of immunoglobulins by newborn calves, a process critical to the survival of newborn mammals, was demonstrated by Balfour and Comline [2] in 1959. This seminal study was later complimented by others demonstrating resorption of intact enzymes. Seifert et al. [24] showed in 1974 that an enzyme contained in pineapples (bromelain) appears in the bloodstream completely intact after oral ingestion.

Karl Hansen [11] must be credited with being the first investigator to have systematically investigated resorption of allergens from the gastrointestinal tract using a modified Prausnitz-Kuestner method [22]. Antibody-containing serum of a patient suffering from milk, fish or egg white allergy is injected subcutaneously into the forearm of the study subjects. The allergen is then presented directly to the gastrointestinal mucosa via a duodenal tube. A hive can be observed at the site of the subcutaneous injection as early as 3 min after presenting the antigen. This scientifically rigorously designed experiment provides proof of concept for resorption and hematogenous spread of biologically intact allergens from the duodenum [12].

Unfortunately, the potential danger of transmitting blood-borne pathogens (human immunodeficiency virus, hepatitis viruses) associated with the injection

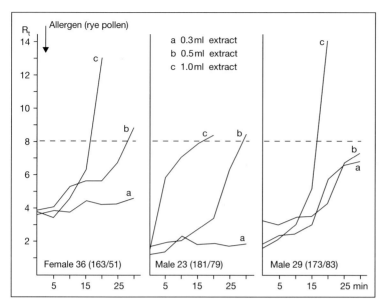

Fig. 5. Reactions of the bronchial system measured by body plethysmography in 3 patients, each given different amounts of allergen extract [15]. Patient figures represent age (years) with the height (cm)/weight (kg) given in parentheses.

of patient serum into a study subject has prevented the use of this technique in more recent times. However, we were able to demonstrate quantitative dose-response curves during oral immunotherapy with pollen allergens using body plethysmographic (R_t) measures of airway obstruction to assess the degree of immune response as figures 4 and 5 show [15].

Most studies have investigated resorption of allergens from the small intestine, whereas little is known about resorption of allergens or other proteins from the large intestine. The large intestine is mainly recognized as the site of resorption of free water, electrolytes, and water-soluble vitamins. However, resorption of streptokinase after rectal application as well as resorption of human albumin from the large intestine have been described [1, 17, 25].

The advent of oral/sublingual immunotherapy has redirected interest towards resorption of allergens from the oral mucosa. The resorption of small nonprotein molecules such as ethanol and nitro preparations from the oral mucosa is well known and the latter is arguably one of the most frequently used pharmacological interventions in clinical medicine. However, Passalacqua (fig. 6) was the first to demonstrate resorption of allergens from the oral and nasal mucosa. *Parietaria* antigen marked with radioactive iodine

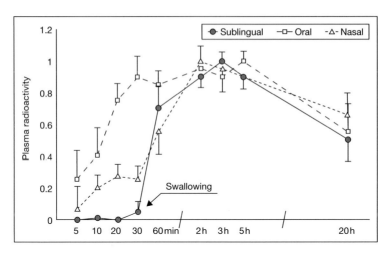

Fig. 6. Plasma radioactivity kinetics (normalized to plasma peak) after administration of radiolabeled allergen by three different routes [20].

was resorbed and appeared in the bloodstream even if remaining in the oral cavity for only 2 min [20].

Oral, sublingual, and nasal application of allergens results in resorption at slightly different rates but peak plasma concentrations are similar with all three applications at 2 h. This difference in early resorption likely has little if any significance in the clinical efficacy of immunotherapy. It is of note that these experiments were undertaken in healthy subjects and it is unknown whether there are similar resorption patterns for allergens in a sensitized patient [21]. Current clinical practice allows swallowing of the allergen solution that has not been resorbed early after sublingual application. Lastly, while of great concern to many, life-threatening complications or anaphylactic reactions have not been reported with oral/sublingual immunotherapy [4, 20].

A review of several standard text books over the past decades reveals a great variety in the assessment of oral immunotherapy ranging from a de facto description of it as clinical practice [5, 27, 28], critical review [6, 27], to rejection [23, 29], or, at worst, a failure to mention it at all [19, 32]. Despite early and conclusive scientific evidence promising success, oral immunotherapy remained a pariah of clinical allergology for a long time. The reader may use this historical review to decide for themselves if and at what time sufficient clinical evidence was available to give our patients broad access to what has only recently become the unequivocal standard of care in the treatment of many allergic diseases.

References

1 Bachmann E: Development of antibodies against perorally and rectally administered streptokinase in man. J Lab Clin Med 1968;72:228–238.

2 Balfour WE, Comline RS: The specifity of intenstinal absorption of large molecules by the newborn calf. J Physiol (Lond) 1959;148:77–78.

3 Bousquet J, Lockey RF, Malling HJ: WHO Position Paper. Allergen immunotherapy: Therapeutic vaccines for allergic diseases. Allergy 1998;53(suppl):44.

4 Bousquet J, Des Roches A, Paradis L, Knani J, Dhivert H, Michel FB: Indications for specific immunotherapy; in Kay AB (ed): Allergy and Allergic Diseases. Oxford, Blackwell, 1997, pp 1234–1242.

5 Bruun E: Specific treatment of bronchial asthma; in Jamar JM (ed): International Textbook of Allergy. Copenhagen, Munksgaard, 1959, pp 271–297.

6 Charpin J: Allergologie, ed 2. Paris, Flammarion, 1986.

7 Curtis HH: The Immunizing Cure of Hay Fever. Med News, New York, 1900, vol 77, pp 16–19.

8 Dakin R: Cited in Tomasi TB Jr: Oral tolerance. Transplantation 1980;29:353–356.

9 Friedländer G: Über die Resorption gelöster Eiweissstoffe im Dünndarm. Z Biol 1896;33: 264–287.

10 Fisher V: Intestinal absorption of viable yeast. Proc Soc Exp Biol 1930/1931;28:948–953.

11 Hansen K: Auslösung der Prausnitz-Küstnerschen Reaktion durch Inhalation des spezifischen Allergens. Proc 1st Int Congr Allergy. Basel, Karger, 1952, pp 999–1002.

12 Hansen K: Über die Resorption von unabgebautem Eiweiss im Dünndarm. 45. Tg Wdtsch Ges Inn Med, Göttingen. Lübeck, Hanse'sches Verlagskontor, 1955, vol 1, pp 34–39.

13 Herbst EFG: Das Lymphgefässsystem und seine Verrichtungen. Göttingen, Vandenhoek & Ruprecht, 1844, pp 333–337.

14 Jorde W, Linskens HF: Zur Persorption von Pollen und Sporen durch die intakte Darmschleimhaut. Acta Allergol 1974;29:165–174.

15 Jorde W, Linsenmann P, Werdermann K, Bohlmann HG: Quantitative Untersuchungen zur enteralen Resorption inhalativer Allergene. Z Immunitätsforsch 1977(suppl 2):135–138.

16 Jorde W: Resorption von Allergenen aus dem Magen-Darm-Trakt. Allergologie 1996;19:569–572.

17 Kremer P, Seifert J: Proteinresorption aus dem Dickdarm; in Seifert J, Ottenjahn R, Zeitz M, Bockemühl J (eds): Ökosystem Darm. Part III. Heidelberg, Springer, 1991, pp 88–95.

18 Marfels F, Moleschott J: Der Übergang kleiner Partikel aus dem Darmkanal in den Milchsaft und das Blut. Wien Med Wochenschr 1854;4:817.

19 Mygind N, Dahl R, Pedersen S, Thestrup-Pedersen K: Essential Allergy, ed 2. Oxford, Blackwell Scientific, 1995.

20 Passalacqua G, Bagnasco M, Mariani G, Falagiani P, Canonica GW: Local immunotherapy: Pharmacokinetics and efficacy. Allergy 1998;53:477–484.

21 Passalacqua G, Villa G, Altrinetti V, Falagiani P, Canonica GW, Mariani G, Bagnasco M: Sublingual swallow or spit? Allergy 2001;56:578.

22 Prausnitz K, Küstner H: Studien zur Überempfindlichkeit. Zentralbl Bakt 1921;86:160–169.

23 Renz H: Spezifische Immuntherapie; in Heppt W, Renz H, Röcken M (eds): Allergologie. Berlin, Blackwell, 1998, pp 152–159.

24 Seifert J, Ganser R, Brendel W: Die Resorption eines proteolytischen Enzyms pflanzlichen Ursprungs aus dem Magen-Darm-Trakt in das Blut und in die Lymphe von erwachsenen Ratten. Z Gastroenterol 1979;17:1–8.

25 Seifert J, Hallfeld K, Figacz G, Eberle B, Brendel W: Modifizierung der Immunantwort durch enteral verabreichtes Proteinantigen. Z Gastroenterol 1979;17:652.

26 Seifert J: Resorption grossmolekularer Substanzen aus dem Magen-Darm-Trakt. Allergologie 1996;19:573–579.

27 Serafini U: Immunologia clinica ed allergologia. Firenze, Uses, 1982, p 1037.

28 Tuft L: Clinical Allergy, ed 2. Philadelphia, Saunders, 1938, p 108.

29 Vaughan WT: Practice of Allergy, ed 2. Saint Louis, Mosby, 1948, p 328.

30 Voit C, Bauer E: Über die Aufsaugung im Dick- und Dünndarm. Z Biol 1869;5:536.

31 Volkheimer G: Das Phänomen der Persorption und seine Bedeutung für allergologische Fragestellungen. Verh Allergie Immunforsch 1966;10:121–125.

32 Wahn U: Die Bedeutung der Hyposensibilisierungs-Behandlung bei Inhalationsallergien; in Wahn U, Seger R, Wahn V (eds): Pädiatrische Allergologie und Immunologie in Klinik und Praxis. Stuttgart, Fischer, 1987, pp 161–169.

33 Wortmann F: Orale Hyposensibilisierung bei inhalationsallergien; in Fuchs E, Schulz KH (eds): Manuale Allergologicum. Deisenhofen, Dustri, 1988, vol 7, 3.3.

Dr. med. Wolfgang Jorde, Internist – Allergologie,
Am Spielberg 38, D–41063 Mönchengladbach (Germany)
Tel. +49 21 61 1 36 55, Fax +49 21 61 20 44 62, E-Mail Wjorde4711@aol.com

Markert UR, Elsner P (eds): Local Immunotherapy in Allergy.
Chem Immunol Allergy. Basel, Karger, 2003, vol 82, pp 33–43

....

Allergen Biodistribution in Humans

Marcello Bagnasco[a], Silvia Morbelli[a,b], Vania Altrinetti[a,b],
Paolo Falagiani[d], Giuliano Mariani[e], Giovanni Passalacqua[c]

[a]Allergy and Clinical Immunology Unit, [b]Nuclear Medicine Unit and
[c]Allergy and Respiratory Diseases Unit, Department of Internal Medicine,
Genoa University, Genoa, [d]Lofarma S.p.A., Milan, and [e]Nuclear Medicine Unit,
Pisa University, Pisa, Italy

Key Words
Immunotherapy · Radiolabelled allergen · Parietaria judaica · Non injective administration · Local immunotherapy

Abstract
Specific immunotherapy performed by noninjectable (oral, nasal or oromucosal) routes was mostly developed in the last 20 years with the main aim to avoid side effects that occasionally occur in the course of injectable immunotherapy. Although evidence of its clinical efficacy has been provided some pharmacokinetics aspects are still to be elucidated. In this review we discuss experimental findings of mucosal processing, biodistribution in healthy or allergic humans of ^{123}I-labelled major allergen of *Parietaria judaica* (the most important cause of seasonal allergy in the Mediterranean area) administered by sublingual or nasal routes. The results available to date show that most allergen administered by mucosal route is absorbed via the gastrointestinal tract; however, a proportion is retained at the mucosal level for a relatively long time. These data are potentially useful to improve immunotherapy treatment protocols by noninjectable routes.

The efficacy of allergen-specific immunotherapy has been largely demonstrated during the last decades, although its action on the immunoregulatory mechanism has been partially elucidated only in recent years [1–7]. The possibility of administering allergen preparations by noninjectable routes has been proposed in the first decades of the 20th century [8, 9]; however, studies concerning noninjectable routes have been developed only over the last 20 years [5, 10–20], with the main aim being to minimize the possibility of severe side effects, which, although only occasionally, have been observed during the course of allergen-specific immunotherapy through injection [21–23].

An allergen preparation has been administered via direct ingestion (oral route) or by so-called 'mucosal' routes: nasal, sublingual or oromucosal. This implies that some local effects or local absorption were expected. As a matter of fact, a demonstration of the clinical efficacy of mucosal allergen immunotherapy has been provided, and some hypotheses about its mechanism of action have been formulated [15–19, 24–32].

However, many points have to be clarified: namely, the mechanism(s) whereby mucosal transit or retention of allergen preparation may exert local or even systemic effects. In fact, these mechanisms are expected to be different depending upon different fate/processing of allergen in contact with different mucosal tissues and their local immune system.

Allergen Handling at the Mucosal Level

Mucosal surfaces are regularly exposed to a wide variety of antigens, including allergens. As a rule, exogenous antigens (and in particular allergens) are expected to be handled by the mucosal immune system in order to clear, at least in part, antigenic challenges before transmucosal absorption and/or to minimize harmful reactions to the organism [33, 34].

As far as specifically allergens are concerned, contact with gastrointestinal or respiratory mucosa appears to deeply modify the systemic response to allergen in experimental animals. In particular IgE response can be reduced or prevented [35–38]. The exact mechanism of such oral 'tolerance' is far from clarified; however, the role of antigen processing and presentation, specifically by dendritic cells, is probably critical [24, 33, 39]. Moreover, systemic changes in immunological reactivity to allergen after sublingual treatment were demonstrated in allergic patients [28], although clear evidence of a T cell shift from Th2 to Th1 response is still lacking [32]. In addition some effects on sublingual immunotherapy on adhesion molecule expression and eosinophil activation have been reported [30, 31]. As far as nasal administration is concerned, a number of data from both animal models and human studies suggest an effect on local immunological phenomena.

Specifically, transmucosal absorption has been observed in experimental animals [40–42]; moreover, the mucosal permeability to macromolecules was reported to be higher in allergic than in normal subjects [42, 43]. In allergic patients, intranasal administration of allergen extracts seems to exert its effect mainly on local clinical manifestations and local immunological response [18]. Thus, local administration of allergen may evoke a 'benign' systemic immunological reaction, or, on the other hand, exert its immunological action locally. The former mainly pertains to the sublingual, the second to the intranasal route.

However, although such a perspective has a well-defined theoretical basis and is supported by experimental evidence, no experimental data have been available until the last few years about the fate of allergens administered locally for immunotherapy in humans, and specifically about local retention/persistence, transmucosal passage, and systemic absorption.

Studies with Radiolabelled Allergen in Healthy Humans

Knowledge of the pharmacokinetics of allergen preparation when locally administered is crucial to understand the mechanism of action of local immunotherapy better and eventually to optimize administration protocols.

Data from animal models are scanty and not easily applicable to humans [40–42]. In the late 1990s an experimental approach has been developed to investigate allergen biodistribution in humans [44]: it involves the use of a purified radiolabelled allergen preparation that is administered by different routes to human volunteers. Scintigraphic imaging was used to follow allergen localization and transit as well as analysis of biological fluid radioactivity.

Such studies have been performed with the major allergen of *Parietaria judaica*, Par j 1. *P. judaica* pollen is one of the most widely diffuse allergen in the Mediterranean area. Par j 1 is a glycoprotein of 12.5 kD molecular weight with 2 tyrosine residues; HPLC-purified preparations were used for labelling with radioactive iodine. The radioactive isotope ^{123}I was chosen due to its favorable emission characteristics; its 139-keV gamma radiation peak is optimal for external detection by the γ-camera. The absence of β-radiation emission and the short half-life (13.2 h) allow minimal exposure when administered in vivo with an absorbed total body radiation dose/experiment of approximately 1/30 of a standard chest x-ray film (administered radioactivity 37/56 MBq ^{123}I). For radiolabelling, the iodo-gene method was used, resulting in a radioactive preparation of adequate specific activity (about 3.7 MBq/μg), with little physical damage of the native molecule and stability to deiodination over several days (as demonstrated in parallel experiments of radiolabelling with ^{125}I, half-life 60 days).

^{123}I-labelled Par j 1 was given to normal volunteers, either sublingually, or orally (direct swallowing of the antigen) or intranasally. The administration schedules and protocols of scintigraphic acquisition and blood sampling are summarized in figure 1. For the sublingual route the dose was delivered in 0.1–0.2 ml under the tongue by a micropipette, then the subject was asked not to move or swallow for 30 min; during this time, a dynamic scintigraphy

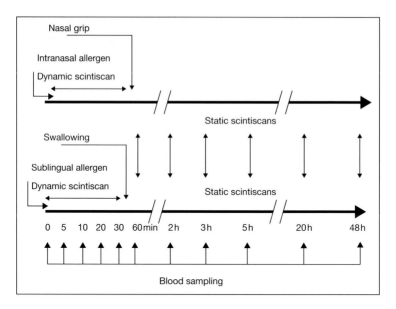

Fig. 1. Study design to investigate allergen pharmacokinetic by [123]I Par j 1 administration.

(1 frame/min) was performed of the mouth region. This protocol was chosen to maximize the time of contact with sublingual mucosa.

Other subjects received the allergen sublingually as above, but were asked to spit it into a container provided for this purpose 3 min later; then a new scintigraphic acquisition was started (sublingual-spit protocol) [45]. When the oral route was used, the radiolabelled allergen was administered in 50 ml water and immediately swallowed. For the intranasal route, the dose was sprayed into a nostril by means of a buffer, exactly as for the nasal therapeutic administration, a nasal grip was immediately applied and a scintigraphic acquisition was performed over 30 min. In all cases (see fig. 1) blood samples were drawn for plasma radioactivity counting and plasma chromatography, and static scintigraphic acquisitions were performed at different times (up to 48 h).

In order to minimize thyroid uptake of free radioactive iodine derived from radiolabelled allergen deiodination, saturated potassium iodide solution was given to the subjects in the 5 days before the study followed by potassium perchlorate for 2 days, starting from the day of the study.

Biodistribution of Radiolabelled Allergen by Sublingual Route

Early scintigraphic imaging during sublingual retention of the radioallergen clearly showed no change in the radioactive content of the mouth before

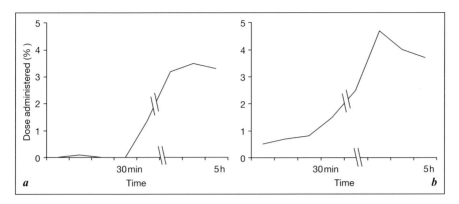

Fig. 2. Plasma radioactivity profiles obtained in 2 healthy volunteers after administration of ^{123}I-Par j 1 by sublingual (*a*) or intranasal (*b*) route, respectively. ^{123}I-Par j 1 was administered at time 0; for sublingual administration the subject swallowed at 30 min. The radioactivity is expressed as percent of the administered dose.

swallowing. This was confirmed by the analysis of plasma radioactivity; in fact, plasma radioactivity was at background levels before swallowing and rapidly increased thereafter (see representative experiment of fig. 2).

After swallowing rapid visualization of the esophagus and stomach was obtained, as in all gastrointestinal transit studies with a radioactive bolus. The small intestine appeared a few minutes after the stomach; then renal excretion and visualization of the urinary bladder took place within about 3 h, as shown by static scintigraphic studies. In the control subjects who immediately swallowed the radioactive allergen, rapid distribution of radioactivity in the gastrointestinal tract was apparent, superimposable to what was observed for the sublingual route after swallowing: plasma radioactivity counts, accordingly, strictly paralleled those recorded for the sublingual route after swallowing.

Interestingly, after sublingual, but not oral administration of radiolabelled allergen, a significant amount of radioactivity (about 2% of the administered dose) persisted at the level of the mouth for up to 20 h, even after extensive mouth rinsing, as shown by late scintigraphic acquisition; in control experiments where free ^{123}I was administered, radioactivity disappeared quickly from the sublingual region.

In subjects where the sublingual/spit schedule was applied, radioactivity recovered in the spat saliva accounted for 30% or less of the administered dose; the remaining radioactivity persisted within the mouth, the gastrointestinal tract was visualized, and plasma radioactivity rose immediately after swallowing, as in the sublingual-swallow protocol. This indicates that rapid distribution of the allergen on oral mucosa occurs following sublingual administration and that the spitting procedure does not substantially affect allergen biodistribution [45].

From these data, a direct absorption of allergen from oral mucosa is apparent; the majority of the radiolabelled allergen is swallowed and processed/absorbed in the gastrointestinal tract. It is likely that the systemic immunological effects observed in previous studies are in most part due to gastrointestinal absorption. As mentioned above, even in sublingual-spit protocols the majority of radiolabelled allergen is transported to the gastrointestinal tract. For the same reasons, the risk of too rapid sublingual allergen absorption does not appear to have an experimental basis. On the other hand, it may be hypothesized that retention of a fraction of the administered allergen within the oral mucosa plays a role in the mechanism of action of sublingual immunotherapy, possibly via handling by the local immune system; in fact, processing of administered allergen by dendritic cells of oral mucosa and presentation to T cells have been shown in experimental models [24, 46].

Biodistribution of Radiolabelled Allergen by Intranasal Route

After radiolabelled allergen inhalation, dynamic scintigraphy showed that a remarkable fraction of radioactivity moved from the nose towards the upper pharynx, probably by mucociliary clearance, was gradually swallowed. The esophagus was visualized, followed by the stomach and gastrointestinal tract (as for oral administration); consistently, plasma radioactivity gradually increased over time starting during the first few minutes. No specific radioactivity accumulation was observed at any time at the level of the bronchial tree. It is worth noting, as observed for sublingual administration, that a persistence of radioallergen at the level of nasal mucosa was observed for as long as 40 h. The retained radioactivity was relatively high (about 10% of the administered dose). Also in this case, control experiments with free ^{123}I inhalation did not result in long-term local radioactivity persistence.

As already observed for sublingual administration, even in this case both local retention and systemic absorption of allergen by intestinal tract are likely to occur, the locally retained fraction being higher. Notably the lack of bronchial deposition of radiolabelled Par j 1 seems to minimize the risk of asthma attacks due to undesired bronchial exposure, as previously discussed [5].

Processing of Locally Administered Allergen

Extensive fragmentation of the allergic extracts has been demonstrated to occur in the duodenum [46, 47], whereas some data suggest partial degradation due to saliva (using the RAST inhibition method) [47]. We evaluated the gel filtration radioactivity profile of saliva after sublingual administration of radio-labelled Par j 1; 0.2 ml of saliva was withdrawn by micropipette from the mouth. The radioactivity profile obtained showed a major peak in the molecular weight region of native allergen, only small fractions of radioactivity being localized in the low molecular weight fractions (fragments, free iodine), as occurs for freshly radiolabelled allergen. Thus, extensive fragmentation of Par j 1 does not seem to occur sublingually [44].

Plasma radioactivity was shown to reach a peak at about 2 h following allergen administration by either the sublingual or intranasal route. Plasma radioactivity gel filtration at 1 and 2 h showed a quite different profile with respect to native allergen, in that only a small fraction of radioactivity was present in the molecular weight region of the intact molecule, whereas the majority was in the low molecular weight region (small peptides and free iodine). This is consistent with extensive deiodination and fragmentation of radiolabelled allergen within the stomach and intestine.

That part of radioactivity in the low molecular weight region which is represented by small molecular fragments, and not only by free iodine, has been demonstrated by ion exchange chromatography; moreover, control individuals assuming free ^{123}I by the sublingual as well as the intranasal route showed a far different plasma radioactivity profile with faster disappearance following the absorption peak. Altogether the available data suggest that the allergen molecule substantially maintains its physical properties during the first mucosal contact, but undergoes extensive degradation within the gastrointestinal tract.

Biodistribution of Radiolabelled Allergen in Allergic Individuals

The above-mentioned results concerning Par j 1 biodistribution were obtained in normal volunteers [44, 45]. In other experiments [48, 49] radio-labelled Par j 1 was administered to volunteers allergic to *P. judaica* by the sublingual or intranasal route. For the sublingual route the preparation was administered in tablets, as in a normal course of immunotherapy; the tablets were kept in the mouth until dissolved, then they were swallowed.

In these experimental conditions too, similar results were obtained; no transmucosal passage of the tracer to the bloodstream before swallowing, as well as local persistence for hours after administration were observed. Accordingly, plasma radioactivity profile and radioactivity gel filtration profile at its peak were similar to the former set of experiments. Preliminary studies were also performed in subjects with allergic rhinitis due to *P. judaica* pollen, receiving radiolabelled Par j 1 intranasally. At variance with what is shown in normal individuals, the disappearance rate of radioactivity from the nasal region was much faster, and accordingly an earlier peak of plasma radioactivity (1 h) was observed. Moreover, no local long-term persistence of radioactivity at the nasal level was apparent. These data may be consistent with a faster transit of allergen to the upper pharynx and esophagus, but also with local transmucosal absorption.

These data, although preliminary, suggest that local allergic inflammation may affect the biodistribution and fate of the administered allergen, in particular by reducing its local persistence.

Chemical Modification of Allergen: Effect on Biodistribution

Chemically modified allergen (allergoids) are frequently used for immunotherapy. We have comparatively evaluated the biodistribution of native radiolabelled Par j 1 and the corresponding monomeric carbamylated allergoid (monoid) [48].

The results obtained showed no substantial difference in the local kinetics between the two radiolabelled preparations. However, plasma radioactivity profiles showed a significantly higher absorption peak for allergoid: the plasma gel chromatography profile of radioactivity at 2 h constantly showed a well defined, although small, peak in the molecular weight region of intact native allergoid.

Thus, chemical modification of allergen preparation may somehow affect its biodistribution, and part of the protein can be absorbed through the gastrointestinal tract with little or no degradation. An increased resistance of the allergoid to gastrointestinal degradation possibly due to substitution of the majority of NH_2 residues, resulting in reduced sensitivity to enzymatic hydrolysis, could explain the higher absorption of allergoid with respect to allergen.

This fact may have a role in the therapeutic action of the allergoid; it is worth noting that the chemical modification does not affect the ability of the allergoid to elicit a specific antibody response against the native allergen [50].

Conclusions

The studies of allergen pharmacokinetics using ^{123}I-labelled allergen preparation proved to be a unique tool to obtain biodistribution data in humans. The information obtained has provided insight about the mechanism of allergen absorption in humans. Different to what was observed in animal studies [40–42], rapid direct sublingual passage to the blood is not apparent. However, local retention is observed with possible involvement of the local immune system. Nasal mucosal persistence is even more consistent. Anyway, systemic absorption of extensively processed allergen occurs with both sublingual and intranasal routes, and systemic effects of immunotherapy are probably mainly related to this fact.

Local allergic inflammation may significantly influence the persistence and/or transmucosal absorption of the allergen, and this may have implications for concomitant pharmacological treatments. Finally, chemical modification of allergen may influence its biodistribution. Nevertheless, it should be noted that the short physical half-life of ^{123}I may make it possible to underestimate the local persistence of radiolabelled allergen, in that scintigraphic evaluation is hardly possible some time (more than 48 h) after tracer administration. Moreover, the chromatographic analysis of plasma radioactivity performed to date does not provide information about the chemical nature or biological activity of allergen fragments.

Perspectives

It is important to note that the data available deal with a single purified allergen (Par j 1) and its chemically modified counterpart. The first aim of future allergen biodistribution research will be to investigate other major pollen or perennial allergens with different chemical and physical properties, to draw more general conclusions. In addition, a more detailed analysis of physical and biological properties of peptide fractions resulting from processing of locally administered allergen (as radioactivity HPLC chromatography and/or RAST inhibition studies) on fractions will be required.

All these experimental data, in addition to contributing to a better understanding of the mechanisms of action of local allergen immunotherapy, may make it possible to better devise treatment protocols and allergen/allergoid preparations for therapeutic use.

References

1 Noon L: Prophylactic inoculation against hay fever. Lancet 1911;1:1572.
2 Rachemann FN, Edwards MC: Asthma in children. A follow-up study on 688 patients after an interval of 20 years. N Engl J Med 1952;246:915–919.
3 Johnstone D: A study of the natural history of bronchial asthma in children. Am J Dis Child 1968; 115:213–221.
4 Johnstone D, Dutton A: The value of hyposensitization therapy for bronchial asthma in children: A 14-year study. Pediatrics 1968;42:793–799.
5 Malling HJ, Weeke B: Immunotherapy. EAACI position paper. Allergy 1993;48(suppl 14):9–30.
6 Abramson MJ, Puy RM, Weiner JM: Is allergen immunotherapy effective in asthma? A meta-analysis of randomized controlled trials. Am J Respir Crit Care Med 1995;151:969–974.
7 Bousquet J, Lockey RF, Malling HJ: Allergen immunotherapy: Therapeutic vaccines for allergic disease. WHO position paper. Allergy 1998;53(suppl 44):1–42.

8   Dunbar WP: The present state of knowledge of hay fever. J Hyg 1913;13:105.
9   Black JH: The oral administration of pollen. J Lab Clin Med 1927;12:1156.
10   Scadding GK, Brostoff J: Low dose sublingual therapy in patients with allergic rhinitis and asthma due to house dust mite. Clin Allergy 1986;16:483–491.
11   Moller C, Dreborg S, Lanner A, Björksten B: Oral immunotherapy of children with rhinoconjunctivitis due to birch pollen allergy. Allergy 1986;41:271–279.
12   Taudorf E, Laursen CL, Lanner A, Björksten B, Dreborg S, Søborg M, Week B: Oral immunotherapy in birch pollen hay fever. J Allergy Clin Immunol 1987;80:153–161.
13   Leng X, Fu YX, Ye ST, Duan SQ: A double blind trial of oral immunotherapy for *Artemisia* pollen asthma with evaluation of bronchial response to pollen allergen and serum specific IgE antibodies. Ann Allergy 1990;64:27–31.
14   Giovane A, Bardare M, Passalacqua G, Ruffoni S, Scordamaglia A, Ghezzi E, Canonica GW: A three years double blind placebo-controlled study with specific oral immunotherapy to *Dermatophagoides*: Evidence of safety and efficacy in pediatric patients. Clin Exp Allergy 1994;24:53–59.
15   Sabbah A, Hassoun S, Le Sellin J, Andre C, Sicard H: A double blind placebo controlled trial by the sublingual route of immunotherapy with a standardized grass pollen extract. Allergy 1994; 49:309–313.
16   Andri L, Senna GE, Betteli C, Givanni S, Andri G, Falagiani P: Local nasal immunotherapy for *Dermatophagoides*-induced rhinitis: Efficacy of a powder extract. J Allergy Clin Immunol 1993; 91:587–596.
17   D'Amato G, Lobefalo G, Liccardi G, Cazzola M: A double-blind placebo-controlled trial of local nasal immunotherapy in allergic rhinitis to Parietaria pollen. Clin Exp Allergy 1995;25: 141–148.
18   Passalacqua G, Albano M, Ruffoni S, Pronzato C, Riccio A, DiBerardino L, Scordamaglia A, Canonica GW: Local nasal immunotherapy to *Parietaria*: Evidence of reduction of allergic inflammation. Am J Respir Crit Care Med 1995;152:461–466.
19   Andri L, Senna GE, Andri G, Dama A, Givanni S, Betteli C, Dimitri G, Falagiani P, Mezzelani P: Local nasal immunotherapy for birch allergic rhinitis with extract in powder form. Clin Exp Allergy 1995;25:1092–1099.
20   Malling HJ, Abreu-Nogueira J, Alvarez-Cuesta E, Alvarez-Cuesta E, Bjorksten B, Bousquet J, Caillot D, Canonica GW, Passalacqua G, Saxonis-Papageorgiou P, Valovirta E: Local immunotherapy. Allergy 1998;53:933–944.
21   Committee on the Safety of Medicines: CSM update: Desensitizing vaccines. Br Med J 1986;293: 948.
22   Greenberg MA, Kaufman CR, Gonzales GE, Rosenblatt CD, Smith LJ, Summers RJ: Late and immediate systemic-allergic reactions to inhalant allergen immunotherapy. J Allergy Clin Immunol 1986;77:865–870.
23   Lockey RF, Benedict LM, Turkeltaub PC, Bukantz SC: Fatalities from immunotherapy. J Allergy Clin Immunol 1987;79:660–677.
24   Van Wilsem EJ, van Hoogstraatn IM, Breve J, Scheper RJ, Kraal G: Dendritic cells of the oral mucosa and the induction of oral tolerance. Immunology 1994;833:128–132.
25   Macatinia SE, Hosken NA, Litton M, Vieira P, Hsieh CS, Culpepper JA, Wysocka M, Trinchieri G, Murphy KM, O'Garra A: Dendritic cells produce IL-12 and direct the development of Th1 cells from naive CD4+ T cells. J Immunol 1995;154:5071–5079.
26   McMenamin C, Holt PG: The natural immune response to inhaled soluble protein antigens involves major histocompatibility complex (MHC) class I-restricted CD8+ T cell-mediated but MHC class II-restricted CD4+ T cell-dependent immune deviation resulting in selective suppression of immunoglobulin E production. J Exp Med 1993;178:889–899.
27   Hasseus B, Dahlgren U, Bergenholtz G, Jontell M: Antigen presenting capacity of Langerhans cells from rat oral epithelium. J Oral Pathol Med 1995;24:56–60.
28   Fanta C, Bohle B, Hirt W, Siemann U, Horak F, Kraft D, Ebner H, Ebner C: Systemic immunological changes induced by administration of grass pollen allergens via the oral mucosa during sublingual immunotherapy. Int Arch Allergy Appl Immunol 1999;120:218–224.
29   La Rosa M, Ranno C, Andre C, Carat F, Tosca MA, Canonica GW: Double-blind placebo-controlled evaluation of sublingual-swallow immunotherapy with standardized *Parietaria*

judaica extract in children with allergic rhinoconjunctivitis. J Allergy Clin Immunol 1999;104: 425–432.

30 Passalacqua G, Albano M, Fregonese L, Riccio A, Pronzato C, Mela GS, Canonica GW: Randomised controlled trial of local allergoid immunotherapy on allergic inflammation in mite-induced rhinoconjunctivitis. Lancet 1998;29:968–973.

31 Purrello-D'Ambrosio F, Gangemi S, Isola S, La Motta N, Puccinelli P, Parmiani S, Savi E, Ricciardi L: Sublingual immunotherapy: A double-blind, placebo-controlled trial with *Parietaria judaica* extract standardized in mass units in patients with rhinoconjunctivitis, asthma, or both. Allergy 1999;29:968–973.

32 Frew AJ, Smith HE: Sublingual immunotherapy. J Allergy Clin Immunol 2001;107:441–444.

33 Holt PG, McMenamin C: Defence against allergic sensitization in the healthy lung: The role of inhalation tolerance. Clin Exp Allergy 1989;19:55–62.

34 Mowat AM: The regulation of immune responses to dietary proteins. Immunol Today 1987;8:93–96.

35 Holt PG, Batty JE, Turner KJ: Inhibition of specific IgE responses in mice by pre-exposure to inhaled antigen. Immunology 1981;42:409–417.

36 Holt PG, Vines J, Britten D: Sublingual allergen administration. I. Selective suppression of IgE production in rats by high allergen doses. Clin Allergy 1988;18:229–234.

37 Swarbrick T, Stokes CR, Soothill JF: Absorption of antigens after oral immunization and the simultaneous induction of specific systemic tolerance. Gut 1979;20:121–125.

38 Holt PG, Britten D, Sedgwick JD: Suppression of IgE responses by antigen inhalation: Studies on the role of genetic and environmental factors. Immunology 1987;60:97–102.

39 Sedgwick JD, Holt PG: Suppression of IgE responses in inbred rats by repeated respiratory tract exposure to antigen: Responder phenotype influences isotype specificity of induced tolerance. Eur J Immunol 1984;8:14–15.

40 Mistrello G, Roncarolo D, Gentili M, Zanoni D, Falagiani P: Modified Par j I allergen from *P. judaica* pollen and its rate of absorption in rats. Immunol Lett 1994;40:31–36.

41 Mistrello G, Rapisarda G, Falagiani P: Detection of IgE-binding activity in serum after intranasal treatment of normal rabbits with *P. judaica* extract. Allergy 1991;46:52–55.

42 Falagiani P, Mistrello G: Pharmacokinetics of allergens after local administration. Allergy 1997;52(suppl 33):17–21.

43 Buckle FG, Cohen AB: Nasal mucosal hyperpermeability to macromolecules in atopic rhinitis and extrinsic asthma. J Allergy Clin Immunol 1975;55:213–221.

44 Bagnasco M, Mariani G, Passalacqua G, Motta C, Bartolomei M, Falagiani P, Mistrello G, Canonica GW: Absorption and distribution kinetics of the major *Parietaria judaica* allergen (Par j 1) administered by noninjectable routes in healthy human beings. J Allergy Clin Immunol 1997;100:122–129.

45 Passalacqua G, Villa G, Altrinetti V, Falagiani P, Canonica GW, Mariani G, Bagnasco M: Sublingual swallow or spit? Allergy 2001;56:578.

46 Einarsson R, Renck B, Taudorf E: In vitro studies of degradation of birch and timothy pollen allergen preparations by human duodenal juice. Allergy 1988;43:469–475.

47 Igea JM, Cuevas M, Lazaro M, Quirce S, Cuesta J: Susceptibility of a grass-pollen oral immunotherapy extract to the saliva and gastric fluid digestive process. Allergol Immunopathol (Madr) 1994;22:55–59.

48 Bagnasco M, Passalacqua G, Villa G, Augeri C, Flamigni G, Borini E, Falagiani P, Mistrello G, Canonica GW, Mariani G: Pharmacokinetics of an allergen and a monomeric allergoid for oro-mucosal immunotherapy in allergic volunteers. Clin Exp Allergy 2001;31:54–60.

49 Passalacqua G, Bagnasco M, Mariani G, Falagiani P, Canonica GW: Local immunotherapy: Pharmacokinetics and efficacy. Allergy 1998;53:477–484.

50 Mistrello G, Brenna O, Roncarolo D, Zanoni D, Gentili M, Falagiani P: Monomeric chemically modified allergens: Immunologic and physicochemical characterization. Allergy 1996;51:8–15.

Prof. Marcello Bagnasco, Department of Internal Medicine,
Genoa University, Viale Benedetto XV 6, I–16132 Genoa (Italy)
Tel. +39 0103537979, Fax +39 0103538604, E-Mail allerlab@unige.it

Markert UR, Elsner P (eds): Local Immunotherapy in Allergy.
Chem Immunol Allergy. Basel, Karger, 2003, vol 82, pp 44–52

....

Therapeutic Procedures of Sublingual Immunotherapy in Clinical Practice

G. Zwacka[a], *U.R. Markert*[b,c]

[a] Children's Hospital, Robert Koch Hospital, Apolda, and
[b] Department of Dermatology and Allergology and
[c] Department of Obstetrics, Friedrich Schiller University, Jena, Germany

---

Key Words
Sublingual immunotherapy · Allergy

Abstract
Clinical practice shows that a number of important measures are required to reach a high efficacy of sublingual immunotherapy. These measures include a specific and exact diagnosis of allergy, a high and reliable compliance of the patient, detailed guidance and explanation by the physician, and a strict monitoring of clinical symptoms and possible side effects. The complex inflammatory situation of the allergic patient, especially concerning the conjunctival, nasal and bronchial mucosa as well as eczema, should be explored in detail and treated with anti-inflammatory medication. After having reviewed the international literature combined with personal practical experience, we interpret and suggest that noninflammatory circumstances increase the chances of success of immunotherapies in allergy; nonetheless, several of these interpretations have not yet been confirmed by clinical studies.

Introduction

This chapter is based on experimental data in combination with experience in clinical practice. Some of the clinical observations and recommendations mentioned have not yet been published. They should be understood as preliminary, and confirmation by clinical studies is desirable.

Various specific antigens induce clinical symptoms in allergic patients by triggering an IgE-dependent immune response. Air-borne allergens are very often implicated in the pathogenesis of acute attacks of allergic rhinitis, asthma, conjunctivitis or atopic eczema. They derive mostly from mite excrements, animal proteins from saliva or skin exfoliation, or are seasonal allergens such as pollen or fungi spores.

We suggest that allergic manifestations, which appear as asthma bronchiale and allergic rhinitis and thereby within the same joint airway system, should be regarded as one single disease [1–3].

The longer a perennial or seasonal allergy exists, the more chronic mucosa disorders arise, which, in slight cases, can be improved or almost normalized with a short-term medication treatment. In more serious cases, for example following a chronic allergic asthma bronchiale, almost irreversible damage of the airways (airway remodelling) develops, which requires treatment with inhalative corticoids for several years in combination with a causal therapy, as far as it may still be promising.

Necessity of Anti-Inflammatory Treatment before and during Sublingual Immunotherapy

The classical IgE-mediated allergic type I reaction is accompanied during the early phase by a mast cell and basophil degranulation and the delivery of preformed or newly synthesized mediators, such as histamine, prostaglandins, leukotrienes, cytokines and others, which provoke the typical symptoms of mucosa swelling, itching, watery secretions, mucosa edema and erythema. During the late phase, chemotactic factors, including prostaglandins, leukotrienes and interleukins, lead to an inflammation induced by eosinophils and their factors, which causes long-lasting destructive inflammatory processes of the nasal and bronchial mucosa.

The supplementary presence of viruses, bacteria, air pollutants or microparticles can further trigger or support such inflammation. Cytotoxic mediators of the late phase of inflammation are additionally responsible for disorders of the mucociliary transport system, epithelial damage and dysfunction of the immunological mucosa defense against viruses and bacteria.

Interleukin-dependent proteins, mostly derived from eosinophils, such as eosinophil cationic protein (ECP) or major basic protein (MBP), play a major role in the upregulation of intercellular adhesion molecules (especially ICAM-1 and ICAM-2, members of the immunoglobulin superfamily) a few minutes following contact with an inflammation-inducing allergen. The increased ICAM-1 expression is detectable on the nasal as well as the bronchial mucosa. Adhesion molecules are important receptors for rhinoviruses, which might be the reason why after very slight exposure of allergic patients to allergens, without notable symptoms, an increased number of virus infections emerge and up to 50% of allergic asthma attacks are correlated with virus infections [5–7].

We suggest that diseases coexisting with allergy, such as conjunctivitis, asthma or atopic eczema, require a simultaneous anti-inflammatory therapy during an outbreak, because active allergic inflammation processes inhibit the induction of tolerance. It might be expected that during an acute or latent allergic inflammation, a local or subcutaneous allergen application leads to a stimulation of this inflammation, but not to tolerance [8].

In atopic eczema, during a state of no tolerance, small quantities of allergens are able to induce T cell activation leading to the activation of an atopic skin manifestation, and also to the induction of allergic mucosa reactions, either immediately or with a delay of several days. Exogenous aeroallergens are absorbed by antigen-presenting cells located in the skin or mucosa and are presented to T cells, which secrete a Th2-favored interleukin profile leading to IgE production. Stimulated T cells returning to skin areas, stimulated Langerhans cells and other dendritic cells of the skin as well as monocytes, eosinophils, basophils and mast cells, which express the high-affinity IgE receptor, are involved in the generation of local inflammation. Allergens, which are absorbed via IgE and the high-affinity IgE receptor, induce a far stronger T cell activation than those which are natively internalized by antigen-presenting cells [9].

Therefore, we emphasize the necessity to forcefully downregulate all allergic inflammation processes before commencing immunotherapy and to continue with such treatment until tolerance towards the allergen has been acquired. Clinical experience very clearly demonstrates that patients receiving anti-inflammatory therapy during both subcutaneous or sublingual immunotherapy (SLIT) have a rapid and stable amelioration of their chronic and relapsing symptoms.

Chemical irritants, for example chlorified water in swimming pools, may lead to chronic nasal congestion during allergic rhinitis in combination with obstruction of the sinuses followed by a secondary bacterial infection or to mucosal edema, which can induce local disorders of oxygenation and headaches [10]. The consequent respiration through the mouth often leads to bronchial obstruction because of a frequently coexisting unspecific bronchial hyperreactivity. Therefore, such irritants should be avoided.

In summary, different results of the therapy may depend not only upon different grading and the previous duration of the allergic disease, but also upon the intercurrent diseases or less evident allergic skin or mucosa inflammation mentioned. Its easy application and few side effects frequently seem to lead to an insufficient monitoring of SLIT patients, where the opposite would be appropriate.

Options for Symptomatic Adjuvant Therapies

Clinical analyses confirmed that topic glucocorticoids as well as most H_1 antihistamines, especially of the 3rd generation, are able to inhibit the upregulation of ICAM-1 on epithelial cells during early and late phases of allergic inflammation [11, 12].

Intranasal or inhalation glucocorticoid therapy reduces the expression of Th2-related interleukins and increases IFN-γ as well as the corresponding receptors [13].

Since histamine is the main mediator of the allergic inflammation during both early and late phases, it is necessary to apply modern selective H1 blockers (for example, ebastine, loratidine or cetirizine) in a parallel way to SLIT. This eliminates minimal persistent inflammation. It becomes evident on the cellular level and can be assessed by the presence of cellular inflammation mediators, interleukins and epithelial expression of adhesion molecules, but without clinical symptoms of allergy [14, 15].

Such adjuvant therapy should be performed for several months after grass or tree pollen exposure and perennially for mite allergy patients; nevertheless, clinical symptoms disappear after mattress and pillow encasing measures. It should be initiated before immunotherapy as well as be continued during immunotherapy, when therapy-related side effects or allergy-related symptoms appear or virus infections of the respiratory tract occur [16, 17].

The adjuvant application of leukotriene antagonists (for example, zafirlukast or montelukast) should be considered especially when allergy persists for several years or when the patient's allergen spectrum is wide. In our experience, a pretreatment of 1–2 months before starting immunotherapy gave positive results.

In case of an obstruction of the nasal airways, the swelling should first be reduced and then the patient should apply the anti-inflammatory medication to ensure its necessary distribution over the complete mucosa. Antihistamines in addition to oral therapy may also be applied locally, intranasally or conjunctivally. The combination of all three substance groups (H_1 antihistamines, topic glucocorticoids and antileukotrienes) as a pretreatment as well as a symptomatic treatment during immunotherapy increases the chances of success of hyposensitization in our experience [unpubl. data].

Skin manifestations of accompanying atopic eczema require a parallel local anti-inflammatory therapy, specifically with topic corticoids, anti-itching preparations and various fatty ointments. In the future, tacrolimus and pimecrolimus preparations might play a special role because they are able to substitute the application of corticoids [18].

Application Methods of SLIT

The most frequently recommended method of applying SLIT is to put it under the tongue and keep it there for 1–2 min and then to swallow it.

Since multiple sensitizations are more frequent than monoallergies, a clear therapeutic strategy concerning a combined immunotherapy is required. It should be analyzed whether different allergens should be applied in one single preparation or separately at different times. In our practice, a longer stay of combined solutions on the mucosa of 3–5 min seems to give promising results.

Beside the quality of allergen solutions and their standardization (µg major allergen/ml), dosage and intervals of application are of great importance, but clinical analyses are still lacking. Based on international experience and several studies, ARIA 2001 recommended a 50- to 100-fold higher dosage for sublingual plus swallow application than for subcutaneous immunotherapy [4, 19–26].

Thus far, only preliminary analyses have been available concerning allergen dosage-dependent mucosal binding and absorption in combination with clinical and immunological efficacy. Bagnasco et al. [27] demonstrated that only 2% of the applied dose were bound to the oral mucosa and remain there for up to 20 h. The results were similar after spitting out or swallowing the preparation. In the stomach and intestines, the marked allergens were fragmented into small peptides and free iodine, while saliva did not induce fragmentation of the major allergen *Parietaria judaica*. After only 10 min of exposure to gastric acid, allergens lose 90% of their allergenicity [28].

Peptides underlie an MHCI and MHCII presentation through the mucosa-associated lymph system of the intestine and are able to stimulate CD8 and CD4 T cells [29]. To discover to what extent they may function as allergens and to estimate the quantity and therapeutic effects of absorbed peptides, further studies will be necessary. To reduce the fragmentation of allergens in the gastrointestinal tract, we recommend applying SLIT after a small meal, which reduces gastric acidity. More than 200 of our patients successfully follow these recommendations.

5 of our patients applied SLIT before brushing their teeth or rinsing their mouth for a duration of 2 years. The symptom scores of these patients concerning their birch and grass pollen allergies were obviously worse than in those patients, who avoided any oral procedures for 90 min after SLIT. We observed a special increase of clinical efficacy, when patients applied SLIT in the evening before sleeping [unpubl. data; our observations]. In this way, a continuous oral mucosal resorption overnight is ensured as well as a lower gastric pepsinogen productivity and acid-induced degradation. Therefore, we suggest that, when two allergens are applied intermittently, the one, whose season is

coming up next, should be given in the evening. Although there are no studies available, we recommend applying up to three different allergen solutions separately at three different time points during the day, whereas four allergen solutions should be combined into two groups with an increased single dose.

In our experiments, we appeared to be unsuccessful in treating only some of the allergies of a polysensitized patient during 1 year and the remaining ones during the following year. The increased susceptibility for new sensitizations induced by preexisting allergies also indicates exacerbating interaction of coexisting sensitizations [30, 31]. Therefore, we assume that inflammatory reactions of nontreated allergies also influence the state of the treated allergy and impair the success of the treatment. We suggest treating all allergies simultaneously, and in severe cases, there should be a parallel application of both SLIT and subcutaneous immunotherapy.

Side Effects of SLIT

Before starting any immunotherapy, the physician should consider the adequate therapy taking into account all the individual circumstances of the patient and advise the patient about the possible success and risks as well as alternative therapies. Although being low, the risk of severe side effects with subcutaneous immunotherapy is much higher than with SLIT and in contrast to the subcutaneous application, no lethal anaphylactic event has been observed with SLIT worldwide. Nevertheless, even with subcutaneous therapy, lethal cases are extremely rare and, especially since allergen standardization is at present much better than it was several years ago, its safety has increased significantly. With SLIT, patients usually only complained about local oral reactions, which were generally described as itching, burning or numbness. Such symptoms were observed in randomized placebo-controlled studies in children as well as in adults [22, 32–34]. Moreover, an isolated or accompanying oral allergy syndrome does not represent a contraindication for SLIT [35].

The most severe side effects, which may occur during SLIT, consist of the allergic symptoms themselves such as allergic rhinitis, asthma attacks or atopic eczema [31]. Anaphylactic reactions are not expected, because allergens do not penetrate the mucosa in an unlimited way, thus entering blood vessels, as is possible after injections.

The physician can obtain a reliable impression of a patient's tendency to develop side effects before starting SLIT by applying 5 drops of the initial dose in the clinic and observing the patient for 30 min.

Following a long period of SLIT application without side effects or during the application of the maintenance dose, the probability that new side effects appear decreases continuously [31]. In some cases, parents complain about the sudden manifestation of such new symptoms, mostly swellings of the tongue or of the cheek mucosa, which persist for 20–30 min. In many cases the reason are mucosal injuries, including necroses induced by teeth braces, carious teeth combined with injuries by the tongue due to continuous manipulation or aphthous stomatitis. Anti-inflammatory mouth washes are able to quickly ameliorate such situations and to eliminate the side effects [our unpubl. observations].

In summary, after evaluation of personal experience together with published data, we recommend that inflammatory processes before and during immunotherapies should be reduced to increase the chances of success of the therapy and to reduce side effects.

Acknowledgment

We thank Justine Fitzgerald for reviewing the English language of our manuscript.

References

1 Grossmann J: One airway, one disease. Chest 1997;111(suppl):11S–16S.
2 Rowe-Jones JM: The link between the nose and lung, perennial rhinitis and asthma: Is it the same disease? Allergy 1997;52:8–20.
3 Vignola AM, Crampette L, Mondain M, Sauvere G, Czarlewski W, Bousquet J, Campbell AM: Inhibitory activity of loratidine on cells. Allergy 1995;50:200–203.
4 Bousquet J, Chanez P, Lacoste JY, White R, Vic P, Michel F-B: Asthma a disease remodelling the airways. Allergy 1992;47:3–11.
5 Jeffry PK, Wardlaw AJ, Nelson FC, Collins JV, Kay AB: Bronchial biopsies in asthma: An ultrastructural, quantitative study and correlation with hyperreactivity. Am Rev Respir Dis 1989; 140:1745–1753.
6 Pattemore PK, Johnston SL, Bardin PG: Virus as precipitants of asthma symptoms. I. Epidemiology. Clin Exp Allergy 1992;22:325–336.
7 Canonica GW: Adhesion molecules in allergy. Role of adhesion molecules in the pathophysiology of allergy. J Investig Allergol Clin Immunol 1997;7:274–276.
8 Wiedermann U, Kraft D: Induction of mucosal tolerance to Bet v 1, the major birch pollen allergen, a review. Allergy Clin Immunol Int 2002;14:17–24.
9 Stingl G, Maurer D: IgE mediated allergen presentation via FcERI on antigen-presenting cells. Int Arch Allergy Immunol 1997;113:24–29.
10 Masieri S, Cavaliere F, Filiaci F: Nasal obstruction improvement induced by topical furosemide in subjects affected by perennial nonallergic rhinitis. Am J Rhinol 1997;11:443–447.
11 Vignola AM, Chanez P, Godard P, Bosquet J: Relationships between rhinitis and asthma. Allergy 1998;53:833–839.
12 Ciprandi G, Ricca V, Passalacqua G, Fasolo A, Canonica GW: Intranasal fluticasone proprinate reduces ICAM-1 on nasal epithelial cells both during early and late phase after allergen challenge. Clin Exp Allergy 1998;28:293–299.
13 Wright ED, Christodoulopoulas P, Small P, Frenkie S, Hamid Q: Th-2 type cytokine receptors in allergic rhinitis and in response to topical steroids. Larnygoscope 1999;109:551–556.

14 Ciprandi G, Buscaglia S, Pesce G, Pronzato C, Ricca V, Parmiani S, Bagnasco M, Canonica GW: Minimal persistent inflammation is present at mucosal level in patients with asymptomatic rhinitis and mite allergy. J Allergy Clin Immunol 1995;96:971–979.

15 Fasce L, Ciprandi G, Pronzato C, Cozzani S, Tosca MA, Grimaldi I, Canonica GW: Cetirizine reduces ICAM-I on epithelial cells during nasal minimal persistent inflammation in asymptomatic children with mite-allergic asthma. Int Arch Allergy Immunol 1996;109:272–276.

16 Fokkens WJ, Godthelp T, Holm AF, Klein JA: Local corticosteroid treatment: The effect on cells and cytokines in nasal allergic inflammation. Am J Rhinol 1998;12:21–26.

17 Ricca V, Landi M, Ferrero P, Bairo A, Tazzer C, Canonica GW, Ciprandi G: Minimal persistent inflammation is also present in patient with seasonal allergic rhinitis. J Allergy Clin Immunol 2000;105:54–57.

18 Meltzer E, Malmstrom K, Lu S, Brenner B, Wie L, Weinstein S, et al: Concomitant montelukast and loratidine as treatment for seasonal allergic rhinitis. Placebo-controlled clinical trail. J Allergy Clin Immunol 2000;105:917–922.

19 Troise C, Voltolini S, Canessa A, Pecora S, Negrini AC: Sublingual immunotherapy in Parietaria pollen-induced rhinitis: A double-blind study. J Investig Allergol Clin Immunol 1995;5:25–30.

20 Clavel R, Bousquet J, Andre C: Clinical efficacy of sublingual-swallow immunotherapy: A double-blind, placebo-controlled trial of a standardized five-grass-pollen extract in rhinitis. Allergy 1998;53:493–498.

21 Bousquet J, Scheinmann P, Guinnepain MT, Perrin-Fayolle M, Sauvaget J, Tonnel AB, Pauli G, Caillaud D, Dubost R, Leynadier F, Vervloet D, Herman D, Galvain S, Andre C: Sublingual-swallow immunotherapy (SLIT) in patients with asthma due to house-dust mites: A double-blind, placebo-controlled study. Allergy 1999;54:249–260.

22 La Rosa M, Ranno C, Andri C, Carat F, Tosca MA, Canonica GW: Double-blind placebo-controlled evaluation of sublingual-swallow immunotherapy with standardized *Parietaria judaica* extract in children with allergic rhinoconjunctivitis. J Allergy Clin Immunol 1999;104: 425–432.

23 Passalacqua G, Albano M, Riccio A, Fregonese L, Puccinelli P, Parmiani S, Canonica GW: Clinical and immunologic effects of a rush sublingual immunotherapy to Parietaria species: A double-blind, placebo-controlled trial. J Allergy Clin Immunol 1999;104:964–968.

24 Purello-D'Ambrosio F, Gangemi S, Isola S, La Motta N, et al: Sublingual immunotherapy: A double-blind, placebo-controlled trial with *Parietaria judaica* extract standardized in mass units in patients with rhiniconjunctivitis, asthma, or both. Allergy 1999;54:968–973.

25 Pajno GB, Morabito L, Barberio G, Parmiani S: Clinical and immunology effects of long-term sublingual immunotherapy in asthmatic children sensitized to mites: A double-blind, placebo-controlled study. Allergy 2000;55:842–849.

26 Bousquet J, Cauvenberge PV, Khaltaev N: Allergic rhinitis and its impact on asthma – ARIA Workshop Report. J Allergy Clin Immunol 2001;108(5 suppl):147–334.

27 Bagnasco M, Mariani G, Passalacqua G, Motta C, Bartolomei M, et al: Absorbtion and distribution kinetics of the major *Paritaria judaica* allergen (Par j 1) administered by noninjectable routes in healthy humans beings. J Allergy Clin Immunol 1997;100:122–129.

28 Igea JM, Cuevas M, Lazaro M: Susceptibility of grass-pollen immunotherapy extract to the salvia and gastric fluid digestive process. Allergol Immunopathol 1994;22:55–59.

29 Blanas E, Davey GM, Carbone FR, Heath WR: A bone marrow-derived APC in the gut-associated lymphoid tissue captures oral antigens and presents them to both CD4+ and CD8+ T cells. J Immunol 2000;164:2890–2896.

30 Silvestri M, Rossi GA, Cozzani S, Pulvirenti G, Fasce L: Age-dependent tendency to become sensitized to other classes of aeroallergens in atopic asthmatic children. Ann Allergy Asthma Immunol 1999;83:335–340.

31 Purello-D'Ambrosio F, Gangemi S, Merendino RA, Isola S, Puccinelli P, Parmiani S, Ricciardi L: Prevention of new sensitizations in monosensitized subjects submitted to specific immunotherapy or not. A retrospective study. Clin Exp Allergy 2001;31:1295–1302.

32 Pradalier A, Basset D, Claudel A, Couturier P, Wessel F, Galvain S, Andre C: Sublingual-swallow immunotherapy (SLIT) with a standardized five-grass-pollen extract (drops and sublingual tablets) versus placebo in seasonal rhinitis. Allergy 1999;54:819–828.

33 Andre C, Vatrinet C, Galvain S, Carat FD, Sicard H: Safety of sublingual-swallow immuno-therapy in children and adults. Int Arch Allergy Immunol 2000;121:229–234.
34 Guez S, Vatrinet C, Fadel R, Andre C: House-dust-mite sublingual-swallow immunotherapy (SLIT) in perennial rhinitis: A double-blind, placebo-controlled study. Allergy 2000;55:369–375.
35 Lombardi C, Passalacqua G, Gargioni S, Berard M: The safety of sublingual immunotherapy in patients with oral allergy syndrome (abstract). Allergy 2000;55(suppl 63):116.

Prof. Dr. Gerhard Zwacka
Kinderklinik, Robert-Koch-Krankenhaus Apolda,
Robert-Koch-Strasse 6/8, D–99510 Apolda (Germany)
Tel. +49 3644 57 12 81, E-Mail sek.paed@rkk-apolda.de

Markert UR, Elsner P (eds): Local Immunotherapy in Allergy.
Chem Immunol Allergy. Basel, Karger, 2003, vol 82, pp 53–61

Efficacy of Sublingual Immunotherapy in Grass Pollen Allergy

Dirk Wessner[a], Jürgen Rakoski[b], Johannes Ring[b]

[a]Private Practice, Stuttgart, [b]Department of Dermatology and Allergology, Technical University Munich, Munich, Germany

Key Words
Sublingual immunotherapy · SLIT · Grass pollen allergy

Abstract
Sublingual immunotherapy (SLIT) was developed to improve the safety of specific immunotherapy; however, its effectiveness is still subject to discussion although the balance sheet for SLIT is improving. In SLIT laboratory parameters and objective measures of allergen reactivity are nonuniform even in studies showing clinical effectiveness, thus subjective symptom scores remain the principal end points. For allergic rhinitis an expert panel collaborating with the WHO recently proposed that SLIT was a viable alternative for injectable immunotherapy (SIT) since a multitude of double-blind placebo-controlled studies had proved the effectiveness of SLIT. Unfortunately, there are only a small number of studies comparing effectiveness of SLIT directly with subcutaneous SIT. These studies demonstrated comparable effectiveness of both therapies. According to the data so far SLIT can be recommended for the therapy of allergic rhinitis in adults and children refusing injectable therapy. For the treatment of allergic asthma both positive and disappointing results have been published. Effectiveness in preventing the onset of allergic asthma in patients with allergic rhinitis has been demonstrated for SIT, while for SLIT this question cannot yet be answered.

Introduction

Sublingual immunotherapy (SLIT) was developed and introduced with the aim to be safer than conventional specific immunotherapy (SIT); this has been demonstrated in two studies [1, 2]. Allergologists are confronted with an increasing number of patients asking for this therapy since the advantages of SLIT for the patient are obvious (no injections, few time-consuming consultations) representing an enormous gain of living quality. In this situation the practising allergologist has to decide whether SLIT is a viable alternative for an individual patient. This review of published data concerning the efficacy of SLIT in grass pollen allergy should give a basis for a scientifically founded recommendation.

As recently stated by the WHO position paper and other consensus papers [3–5] SLIT may be a viable alternative to injectable SIT in patients with allergic rhinoconjunctivitis. The efficacy of SLIT was demonstrated in a multitude of double-blind placebo-controlled studies. However, there are still questions open to discussion. Is SLIT as effective as subcutaneous SIT? Unfortunately there are only a limited number of studies comparing the efficacy of SLIT directly with injectable SIT [6–9]. These studies will be subject to a closer survey. Is SLIT as effective in allergic asthma as in allergic rhinoconjunctivitis? Effectiveness of SLIT in allergic asthma still has to be shown [10]. Furthermore, the preventive effect of SLIT should be looked at. This article will present and discuss the data available concerning effectiveness of SLIT in grass pollen allergy.

Parameters to Control Effectiveness

To determine effectiveness of SLIT various parameters were measured. Most often clinical symptom and medication scores or combinations of the two were used as parameters of effectiveness. In grass pollen allergy allergen challenges were rarely performed in controlled studies; only one study performed a nasal provocation test [11] and one other study performed peak nasal inspiratory flow measurement, a titrated skin prick test, and a conjunctival provocation test [12]. In these studies no significant reduction of allergen reactivity to grass pollen was detected compared with placebo treatment. Immunological changes were investigated in five studies [6, 11–15]. According to the Th2/Th1-swift theory immunotherapy should effect an immunological change shown as a marked decrease of the allergen-specific IgE/IgG4 ratio. However, only in three out of five studies a significant decrease of the IgE/IgG4 ratio was demonstrated and even in these publications no correlation with clinical improvement was found (investigated in two studies [11, 14]). One study investigated immunological changes during SLIT with grass pollen without the assessment of clinical parameters [16]. The SLIT-spit method was performed for 1 year with a cumulative allergen dose of approximately 80 µg of major allergen. A significant increase of specific IgG and IgG4 antibodies was found.

However, the IgE/IgG4 ratio did not change and Th1/Th2 T cell clones, established from the peripheral blood of the patients, did not change during SLIT. The lymphoproliferative response of T cells showed a significant decrease in reactivity to grass pollen extract (p = 0.001). In two studies directly comparing SLIT with injectable SIT a statistically significant increase of allergen-specific IgG and IgG4 was demonstrated only for injectable SIT but not for SLIT [6, 8]. Since even in subcutaneous SIT no individual correlations between immunological changes and clinical effectiveness exist, changes of immunological parameters may be an indicator for immunological reactivity but not for clinical effectiveness. Therefore, to prove clinical efficacy immunological parameters are of limited use and clinical parameters such as symptom and medication scores must be studied.

Allergic Rhinoconjunctivitis

Efficacy of SLIT in allergic rhinoconjunctivitis due to grass pollen has been assessed in many controlled studies [6, 11–15, 17, 18] shown in table 1. The study designs included studies with preseasonal as well as with coseasonal treatment. The number of studied patients ranged from 20 to 136. All but two studies surveyed adults. The study design was double-blind in all except two studies [12, 13]. All of these studies reported clinical benefits shown by a significant reduction of symptom or medication scores. In the open study of Gozalo et al. [12] patients were treated preseasonally for 6 months with two thirds of patients in the verum group and one third of patients in the control group. No coseasonal therapy was administered, reaching a cumulative allergen dose of 250 biological units (BU). Symptom and medication scores were assessed for a period of 12 weeks during the pollen season. Comparison of the symptom scores during the first year showed no significant differences; however, consumption of drugs – principally of nasoocular drugs – was significantly higher in the control group (p < 0.05). The open study of Feliziani et al. [13] used a so-called 'rush' SLIT regimen reaching the maintenance dose after 30 increasing steps taking the drops twice daily only on 3 days a week under clinical supervision in a hospital. The drops had to be spat out. Maintenance therapy consisted of an application of 10 BU of grass pollen mix sublingually at home only 3 times a week. The difference in scores between the verum and placebo group showed a significant reduction of symptom scores (p < 0.01) and medication scores (p < 0.001). The study with the highest number of patients (n = 136) was published by Clavel et al. [14]. A high-dose SLIT was performed from January to the end of July with a high cumulative allergen dose of 2.6 mg timothy pollen major allergen Phl p 5. During a 14-week period

Table 1. Efficacy of SLIT in grass pollen allergy

Author	Patient No.	Duration	Clinical scores of rhinitis	Medical score	Challenge	IgE/IgG4 ratio
Sabbah et al. [17]	58	17 weeks	$p < 0.05$	$p < 0.01$	n.d.	n.d.
Quirino et al. [6]	20	12 months	$p = 0.002$	$p = 0.002$	n.d.	n.s.
Feliziani et al. [13] (open study!)	20	2 years	$p < 0.01$	$p < 0.001$	n.d.	n.s.
Feliziani et al. [18]	34	one season	$p = 0.01$	$p = 0.002$	n.d.	n.d.
Clavel et al. [14]	136	7 months	n.s.	$p < 0.01$	n.d.	$p < 0.001$
Gozalo et al. [12]	54	12 months	n.s.	$p < 0.05$	n.s.	n.s.
Hordijk et al. [15]	57	10 months	$p < 0.03$	n.s.	n.d.	$p < 0.002$
Pradalier et al. [19]	126	5 months	n.s.	n.s.	n.d.	n.d.
Wessner et al. [11]	32	24 months	n.s.	$p = 0.017$	n.s.	$p < 0.05$

n.d. = Not done; n.s. = not significant.

during the pollen season the medication score was significantly lower in the verum group ($p < 0.02$) compared with the placebo group while the total score of rhinitis and conjunctivitis did not differ significantly between the groups. Another double-blind, placebo-controlled study was performed in the Netherlands [15] with 57 patients over a period of 10 months (January to November). The allergen dose was increased during a 3-week period followed by a twice weekly maintenance dosage of 9,500 BU. Symptom scores were significantly lower in the verum group ($p < 0.03$) while the medication score was similar in both groups. Sabbah et al. [17] studied 58 patients during a 17-week controlled trial in patients with rhinoconjunctivitis due to grass pollen. They found a significant reduction of symptom ($p < 0.01$) and medication scores ($p < 0.01$) in the verum group. In 1995 a double-blind study was published by Feliziani et al. [18] using almost the same treatment schedule except an increase of the top allergen dose of 100% (100 BU/ml). For evaluation of symptom and medication scores only 1 month with the highest grass pollen counts was analyzed. They found a significant reduction of rhinoconjunctivitis symptoms ($p = 0.01$) and a highly significant reduction of drug consumption for rhinoconjunctivitis symptoms ($p = 0.002$). One study used tablets for the application of SLIT; this French multicenter study [19] was performed with 126 patients including 17 children (aged 7–15 years). Allergen application of SLIT consisted of a 15-day progression with drops followed by a once daily administration of a single tablet. The cumulative allergen dose was 0.935 mg of Phl p 5. Assessing the symptom scores no significant reduction of rhinitis symptoms (sneezing, rhinorrhea, nasal itching, nasal obstruction) was found but an improvement of ocular symptoms ($p < 0.05$). The medication score showed no significant difference between the two groups while the use of inhaled salbutamol was significantly lower in the actively treated group ($p < 0.01$). In our own study [11] symptom scores and medication scores were analyzed in 25 patients, finding a significantly lower medication score ($p = 0.017$) with an insignificant reduction of symptom scores while a significant global benefit of the verum therapy was demonstrated ($p = 0.029$). However, objective measurement with the nasal provocation test revealed no significant improvement of allergen tolerance.

Corresponding to most published studies of SLIT with other allergens SLIT with grass pollen demonstrated a fairly consistent benefit as regards symptom or medication scores. Objective measures of allergen reactivity do not generally change. SLIT appears to work in adults as well as in children and seems to be safe. According to the data available SLIT is safer than subcutaneous SIT [1, 2]. However, severe side effects are possible [2].

Efficacy of SLIT versus Subcutaneous SIT

To prove the effectiveness of SLIT placebo-controlled studies are vital. Having demonstrated efficacy, a comparison of SLIT with injectable SIT is crucial for the practising allergologist. Four studies compared SLIT with subcutaneous SIT. All four studies demonstrated comparable efficacy of SLIT with injectable SIT. The double-dummy, double-blind study by Quirino et al. [6] compared SLIT versus injectable SIT in grass pollen-allergic patients ($n = 20$). Therapies were performed for 12 months, with a 2.4-fold higher cumulative allergen dose in SLIT compared with subcutaneous SIT. They found that sublingual and injectable therapy were equally effective according to subjective clinical parameters. A highly significant decrease of symptom scores was found ($p = 0.002$ in SLIT and injectable SIT) as well as in medication scores ($p = 0.0039$ in injectable SIT and $p = 0.002$ in SLIT). There is no control group receiving placebo only. Placebo was used for the double-dummy design only. Therefore, the influence of seasonal grass pollen variations cannot be estimated. The recent double-dummy, double-blind, controlled study by Khinchi et al. [7] investigated the efficacy and safety of SLIT swallow and injectable SIT with birch pollen allergen. The cumulative dose of Bet v 1 was about 210 times higher in SLIT compared with injectable SIT (14,760 vs. 70 μg). Compared with placebo both therapies showed a significantly reduced total score of rhinoconjunctivitis, conjunctivitis, rhinitis and medication intake during the pollen season of the first treatment year. They found no significant difference in symptom and medication scores between the two groups.

However, in the second year due to low pollen counts no significant differences were found between SLIT, injectable SIT, and placebo treatment. Therefore, for judgement of efficacy in such studies pollen counts are inevitable. The open study by Bernardis et al. [8] compared SLIT with injectable SIT in *Alternaria tenuis*-allergic patients (n = 23). An improvement of clinical symptoms was found with both therapies and specific nasal provocation had a statistically significant difference in favor of SLIT. A Swiss study [9] investigated the efficacy of SLIT versus subcutaneous SIT to pollen allergens after 3 years of treatment in 375 patients (aged 18–60 years) with tree and/or grass pollen allergy. A yearly postseasonal evaluation of symptom and drug consumption was done. After 3 years, there were neither statistical differences in the efficacy between the two treatment groups nor in the number of adverse reactions; however, the latter were significantly less severe in the SLIT group. Since only one of these double-dummy studies had a placebo-controlled study design [7] more conclusive data are necessary before SLIT can be recommended for routine treatment instead of injectable SIT.

Cumulative Allergen Dose

Controversy still remains with respect to the dose of SLIT. The optimal therapeutic target dose has still not been fully characterized. It has been demonstrated that antigen concentrations can modulate interleukin-4 production by CD4+ T cells, finding lower IL-4 production [20] and increased INF-γ production [21] after high-dose antigen stimulation of allergen-specific human T cell clones. According to these in-vitro results application of high allergen doses in SLIT seems to be recommended. After application of the allergen by the sublingual route about 2% of the dose persist up to 20 h in the oral cavity according to the findings of Bagnasco et al. [22] who studied the pharmacokinetic of ^{123}I-radiolabelled *Parietaria judaica* major allergen. This finding may add weight to the hypothesis that allergen can gain access to dendritic cells (Langerhans cells) within the sublingual mucosa. When only about 2% of applied allergen can interact with dendritic cells of the oral mucosa this might indicate that for the initiation of immunomodulation high doses of allergen are necessary in SLIT. Actual guidelines [3–5] demand a high-dose therapy in SLIT. According to a WHO position paper [3] the cumulative allergen dose should be up to 20 times higher compared with injectable SIT. In contrast to this recommendation doses at least 50–100 times higher than those used for subcutaneous immunotherapy should be used in SLIT according to the pocket guide of the ARIA expert panel published in 2001. These apparent contradictions might be due to the fact that different commercially available solutions of injectable SIT preparations show great differences in the amount of allergen. Therefore, it is desirable that the cumulative allergen dose for SLIT will be defined as standardized in micrograms of major allergen instead of a variety of ratios comparing the allergen doses in SLIT with antigen doses in various subcutaneous SIT preparations. Furthermore, in contrast to these recommendations of 20- to 100-fold higher allergen doses a comparable efficacy of SLIT with injectable SIT was demonstrated in the double-blind, double-dummy study by Quirino et al. [6] using SLIT with only 2.4-fold greater doses compared with those in injectable therapy. These findings are in good agreement with the results of Bernardis et al. [8] who studied the effectiveness of SLIT versus injectable SIT using only 4-fold greater cumulative allergen doses in SLIT compared with subcutaneous SIT.

Allergic Asthma

Studies investigating effectiveness of SLIT in grass pollen-induced allergic asthma reported a clinical improvement [12, 14, 18]. In all these publications patients with allergic rhinoconjunctivitis were studied with a certain number of patients suffering from allergic asthma. The number of studied patients with asthmatic symptoms was therefore small and sometimes the exact proportion of patients with asthma was indistinct [18]. In the latter study a significant difference for asthmatic symptoms ($p = 0.026$) and drug consumption for asthmatic symptoms ($p = 0.049$) was found when analyzing 1 month with the highest grass pollen count. Also the study of Gozalo et al. [12] found lower scores of respiratory symptoms (34.0 vs. 45.9) and bronchial medication (3.5 vs. 7.6) in the verum group. Significance, however, was only calculated for the overall drug consumption finding a significant improvement, while overall symptom scores showed no significant improvement. Clavel et al. [14] found in the SLIT group only 1 out of 10 patients with previous asthma symptoms suffering from an asthma attack compared to 8 out of 16 patients in the placebo group ($p < 0.02$) at the peak of the pollen season. However, the number of studied patients with asthma was small ($n = 26$) compared with the number of patients included ($n = 136$). The consumption of betamethasone was not studied for asthma patients only. They found an overall significant difference compared with placebo treatment ($p < 0.05$) in favor of SLIT. Unfortunately none of these studies with grass pollen allergens performed bronchial allergen challenge.

SLIT studies focusing more on effectiveness in allergic asthma were done with house dust mites [23–27]. Three of these studies reported a significant improvement of clinical symptoms [24, 26, 27] while one study failed to disclose any statistical significant improvement of asthma symptom scores and treatment scores after 11 and 25 months [25]. Except in one study [28] bronchial allergen challenge showed no significant improvement [25–27]. Also there are still not enough data available to estimate the potential of SLIT to prevent the onset of asthmatic symptoms in patients suffering from allergic rhinoconjunctivitis, while this has already been demonstrated for subcutaneous SIT [29]. Therefore, more and larger controlled clinical trials with SLIT in allergic asthma are useful, although there seem to be no theoretical reasons to doubt its potential [30].

References

1   André C, Vatrinet C, Galvain S, Carat F, Sicard H: Safety of sublingual-swallow immunotherapy in children and adults. Int Arch Allergy Immunol 2000;121:229–234.
2   Lüderitz-Püchel U, Keller-Stanislawski B, Haustein D: Risk reevaluation of diagnostic and therapeutic allergen extracts. An analysis of adverse drug reactions from 1991 to 2000. Bundes-gesundheitsbl Gesundheitsforsch Gesundheitsschutz 2001;44:709–718.
3   Bousquet J, Lockey R, Malling H-J: Allergen immunotherapy: Therapeutic vaccines for allergic diseases. A WHO position paper. J Allergy Clin Immunol 1998;102:558–562.
4   Bousquet J, Malling H-J, Abreu-Nogueira J, Alvarez-Cuesta E, et al: EAACI/ESPACI position paper on local immunotherapy. Allergy 1998;53(suppl 44):1–42.
5   Van Cauwenberge P, Bachert C, Passalacqua G, Bousquet J, Canonica GW, Durham SR, Fokkens WJ, Howarth PH, Lund V, Malling H-J, Mygind N, Passali D, Scadding GK, Wang DY: Consensus statement on the treatment of allergic rhinitis. Allergy 2000;55.116–134.
6   Quirino T, Iemoli E, Siciliani E, Parmiani S, Milazzo F: Sublingual versus injective immuno-therapy in grass pollen allergic patients: A double blind (double dummy) study. Clin Exp Allergy 1996;26:1253–1261.
7   Khinchi MS, Poulsen LK, Carat F, André C, Malling HJ: Clinical efficacy of sublingual-swallow and subcutaneous immunotherapy in patients with allergic rhinoconjunctivitis due to birch pollen. A double-blind, double-dummy placebo-controlled study. Allergy 2000;54(suppl 63):24.
8   Bernardis P, Agnoletto M, Puccinelli P, Parmiani S, Pozzan M: Injective versus sublingual immunotherapy in *Alternaria tenuis* allergic patients. J Investig Allergol Clin Immunol 1996;6: 55–62.
9   Corthay P, Gumowski PI, Bodmer R, Clot B: Efficacy of sublingual versus subcutaneous immunotherapy to pollen allergens after 3 consecutive years of treatment. Annual Meeting of the Swiss Society for Allergology and Immunology, 1996.
10 Rakoski J, Wessner D: A short assessment of sublingual immunotherapy. Int Arch Allergy Immunol 2001;126:185–187.
11 Wessner DB, Wessner S, Möhrenschlager M, Rakoski J, Ring J: Efficacy and safety of sublingual immunotherapy in adults with allergic rhinoconjunctivitis: Results after 2 years of a controlled trial (abstract). Allergy 2001;56(suppl 68):88.
12 Gozalo F, Martin S, Rico P, Alvarez E, Cortes C: Clinical efficacy and tolerance of two year *Lolium perenne* sublingual immunotherapy. Allergol Immunopathol (Madr) 1997;25/5:219–227.
13 Feliziani V, Marfisi RM, Parmiani S: Rush immunotherapy with sublingual administration of grass allergen extract. Allergol Immunopathol (Madr) 1993;21/5:173–178.
14 Clavel R, Bousquet J, André C: Clinical efficacy of sublingual-swallow immunotherapy: A double-blind, placebo-controlled trial of a standardized five-grass-pollen extract in rhinitis. Allergy 1998;53:493–498.
15 Hordijk GJ, Antvelink JB, Luwema RA: Sublingual immunotherapy with a standardized grass pollen extract; a double-blind placebo-controlled study. Allergol Immunopathol (Madr) 1998; 26/5:234–240.

16   Fanta C, Bohle B, Hirt W, Siemann U, Horak F, Kraft D, Ebner H, Ebner C: Systemic immuno-logical changes induced by administration of grass pollen allergens via the oral mucosa during sublingual immunotherapy. Int Arch Allergy Immunol 1999;120:218–224.

17   Sabbah A, Hassoun S, Le Sellin J, André C, Sicard H: A double blind placebo controlled trial by the sublingual route of immunotherapy with a standardized grass pollen extract. Allergy 1994; 49:309–313.

18   Feliziani V, Lattuada G, Parmiani S, Dall'Aglio PP: Safety and efficacy of sublingual rush immunotherapy with grass allergen extracts: A double blind study. Allergol Immunopathol 1995; 23:173–178.

19   Pradalier A, Basset D, Claudel A, Couturier P, Wessel F, Galvain S, André C: Sublingual-swallow immunotherapy (SLIT) with a standardized five-grass-pollen extract (drops and sublingual tablets) versus placebo in seasonal rhinitis. Allergy 1999;54:819–828.

20   Secrist H, Dekruyff R, Umetsu DT: Interleukin 4 production by CD4+ T cells from allergic individuals is modulated by antigen concentration and antigen-presenting cell type. J Exp Med 1995;181:1081–1089.

21   Carballido JM, Carballido-Perrig N, Terres G, Heuser CH, Blaser K: Regulation of the cytokine production of allergen-specific human T-cell clones by the allergen. Int Arch Allergy Immunol 1992;99:366–369.

22   Bagnasco M, Mariani G, Passalacqua G, Motta C, Bartolomei M, Falagiani P, Mistrello G, Canonica GW: Absorption and distribution kinetics of the major *Parietaria judaica* allergen (Par j 1) administered by noninjectable routes in healthy human beings. J Allergy Clin Immunol 1997;100:122–129.

23   La Rosa M, Ranno C, André C, Carat F, Tosca MA, Canonica GW: Double-blind placebo-controlled evaluation of sublingual-swallow immunotherapy with standardized *Parietaria judaica* extract in children with allergic rhinoconjunctivitis. J Allergy Clin Immunol 1999;104:425–432.

24   Pajno GB, Morabito L, Barberio G, Parmiani S: Clinical and immunologic effects of long-term sublingual immunotherapy in asthmatic children sensitized to mites: A double-blind, placebo-controlled study. Allergy 2000;55:842–849.

25   Bousquet J, Scheinmann P, Guinnepain MT, Perrin-Fayolle M, Sauvaget J, Tonnel AB, Pauli G, Caillaud D, Dubost R, Leynadier F, Vervloet D, Herman D, Galvain S, André C: Sublingual-swallow immunotherapy (SLIT) in patients with asthma due to house-dust mites: A double-blind, placebo-controlled study. Allergy 1999;54:249–260.

26   Hirsch T, Sähn M, Leupold W: Double-blind placebo-controlled study of sublingual immunother-apy with house dust mite extract (D.pt.) in children. Pediatr Allergy Immunol 1997;8:21–27.

27   Bahceciler NN, Isik U, Barlan IB, Basaran MM: Efficacy of sublingual immunotherapy in children with asthma and rhinitis: A double-blind, placebo-controlled study. Pediatr Pulmonol 2001;32:49–55.

28   Tari MG, Mancino M, Monti G: Efficacy of sublingual immunotherapy in patients with rhinitis and asthma due to house dust mite: A double blind study. Allergol Immunopathol 1990;18: 277–284.

29   Ross RN, Nelson HS, Finegold I: Effectiveness of specific immunotherapy in the treatment of asthma: A meta-analysis of prospective, randomized, double-blind, placebo-controlled studies. Clin Ther 2000;22:329–341.

30   Holt PG, Sly PD, Smith W: Sublingual immunotherapy for allergic respiratory disease. Lancet 1998;28:613–614.

Dr. med. Dirk Wessner
c/o Hautarztpraxis Dr. Leitz, Marienstrasse 1, D–70178 Stuttgart (Germany)
Tel. +49 711 294092, Fax +49 711 2237246

Markert UR, Elsner P (eds): Local Immunotherapy in Allergy.
Chem Immunol Allergy. Basel, Karger, 2003, vol 82, pp 62–76

······················

Efficacy of Desensitization via the Sublingual Route in Mite Allergy

Stéphane Guez

Unité des Maladies Allergiques, Hôpital Pellegrin-Tripode, Bordeaux, France

Key Words

Sublingual immunotherapy · House dust mite · Desensitization · Asthma · Rhinitis

Abstract

Desensitization via the sublingual route when treating mite allergy is a new technique in immunotherapy that has aroused the interest of an increasing number of allergists. Assessing its effectiveness is difficult because of the multiplicity of the criteria used by the various published studies to determine what constitutes an improvement. But a critical analysis of the results obtained in the various methodologically rigorous studies suggests that treatment is effective when compared to a placebo. It remains, however, necessary to determine whether or not the sublingual route is superior to the subcutaneous route; its ease of use and harmlessness should not be the only criteria when deciding upon a treatment that above all else should be curative.

Desensitization, or specific immunotherapy, fascinates and will continue to fascinate allergologists, particularly since every day, fundamental immunological data produce new and convincing arguments as to the usefulness of this treatment in the early management of allergic conditions [1]. However, the route by which this desensitization is administered is still under study, and it is sometimes difficult to obtain a clear view of the true efficacy of different methods. We shall therefore try to make as objective an assessment as possible, and start by emphasizing the difficulties encountered in assessing the efficacy of these treatments because of the complexity of allergic diseases. After a brief discussion of the different studies concerned, we shall focus only on those done in a double-blind fashion versus placebo and discuss their results and findings which may be of value in everyday practice.

A Few Thoughts on the Notion of the Efficacy of Specific Sublingual Desensitization in Mite Allergy

What Do Allergologists Consider to Be an Effective Treatment?
What Are the Expected Benefits?

At present, no definition exists of what an effective treatment must achieve, and even less of what constitutes effective specific immunotherapy, which probably helps to explain the problems encountered in demonstrating treatment efficacy and how easy it is to criticize clinical studies, which are thus always imperfect or open to improvement. This can be explained by the fact that ideas on disease evolve, with therapeutic objectives changing as our fund of knowledge increases. Thus, for example, although lowering blood pressure values may in the past have seemed a good criterion for the efficacy of antihypertensive therapy, new treatments are now expected to prevent stroke as well! The drop in blood pressure, therefore, only constitutes an intermediate criterion, and the reduction of stroke has become the principal end point. What is the situation regarding specific immunotherapy, and particularly the treatment of mite allergy? The problem is complicated from the start by the multiplicity of symptoms possible with this condition, such as conjunctivitis, rhinitis, or asthma. It is, therefore, necessary to fix the target for efficacy: the disappearance of mite allergy, i.e. all symptoms caused by exposure to this allergen? Or just an improvement in one or more aspects of this allergy, with a reduction in symptom and/or medication scores in the pathology considered? A change in the atopic terrain with a reduction in the number of subsequent sensitizations necessary? A further clinical improvement by comparison with the treatments normally prescribed in line with consensus recommendations in asthma and rhinitis? Or mainly a change of the biological parameters of allergy, indicative of an immune process (IgE and IgG), which in principle should be beneficial?

With What Should Sublingual Desensitization Be Compared?

Having thus chosen one or preferably several criteria to judge efficacy, it is also necessary to discuss the element which will serve as a reference to assess this efficacy. All studies compare desensitization with a placebo: this is evidently necessary to demonstrate that the treatment has a true, immunological action, but should the best efficacy end point not be a comparison with the elimination of the allergen? Indeed, elimination is the first measure recommended when managing an allergic disorder, and the only one which can definitively cure a patient if it is correctly applied [2]. By taking no account of this elimination, studies versus placebo are then limited to considering desensitization as a means of allowing the patient to tolerate a 'normal' dose of mites in his or her environment: the efficacy end point is then no longer an improvement but an absence of reaction to more or less high concentrations of mites in the environment. However, after specific immunotherapy, even if there is no improvement on a daily basis, the demonstrated absence of allergic 'crises' in the presence of a higher concentration of mites should be considered as a therapeutic success!

The most simple method should above all consist in comparing sublingual desensitization with subcutaneous desensitization only, taking into account that the latter has widely proved its efficacy. However, the fact that this efficacy is not recognized by everyone further complicates studies, as not only is it necessary to demonstrate the efficacy or lack of it of desensitization to mites via the sublingual route, but it is also necessary to demonstrate the principle itself of desensitization, using the administration via the sublingual route.

What Is an Effective Treatment for the Patient?

Immunotherapy is designed for a specific patient; it is therefore useful to approach the problem from his or her point of view. However, the demands of patients differ considerably depending on their age and symptoms, and their efficacy criteria may diverge markedly from those of the physician; this may explain the apparent contradictions in studies between objective criteria improved by desensitization and subjective criteria which remain unchanged. Who should we believe? The patient? Who has not had to struggle with an allergic patient in a clinic demanding his injection of sustained-release triamcinolone to relieve incapacitating allergy, because no other treatment provides as much relief? We must therefore be sure that the patient has clearly understood the aims of the treatment and the significance of the parameters chosen to assess its value. Another criteria is safety: an effective treatment must also be safe, or in other words, the harm it may cause must be much less than that resulting from the natural course of the disease under treatment.

As a result, all studies must be discussed, as none alone can answer all these questions and meet all the objectives. We shall therefore review all the studies published concerning sublingual desensitization to mites, and discuss the contribution each has made to answering questions on the efficacy or its absence of this treatment in the management of patients allergic to these organisms.

Analytical Review of Different Studies

Methodology

We only focused on studies complying with WHO (World Health Organization) [3] standards, i.e. performed double-blind versus placebo, using only the sublingual route with mite extracts.

For each study we specified the type of clinical study performed, the number of patients included, the duration of the study, its criteria for their inclusion, the methods employed to study the mite content of the environment when it was carried out (table 1), the therapeutic agents employed and the type of maintenance dose (table 2), the criteria chosen to assess the efficacy of sublingual desensitization, the results and adverse effects observed (table 3).

Study Conducted by Tari et al. [4]

This double-blind, placebo-controlled study included 58 children aged between 5 and 12 years: 30 received sublingual desensitization and 28 a placebo for 18 months. The criteria for inclusion were rhinitis and asthma having progressed for at least 3 years. The criteria used to assess efficacy were based on the results of skin tests, symptom and medication scores, nasal inspiratory peak flow, nasal challenge test, nonspecific methacholine bronchial challenge test, assay of IgG (G1 and G4) specific to mites and the levels of T cells CD4 and CD8.

Results. There was a significant reduction (p < 0.01) in the diameter of papulae in the treated group, with an improvement in the nasal peak flow (p < 0.05), in the specific nasal challenge test (p < 0.01), and in specific and nonspecific bronchial challenge tests. The symptom score was also improved in the treated group regarding rhinitis and asthma, particularly at the end of the study (p < 0.001), but not regarding conjunctival symptoms. More than half of the patients in the treated group also had a 20% or more reduction in the consumption of medication (no statistical calculation). In the treated group there was a significant elevation of specific IgG levels, with an IgG4/IgG1 ratio >1. Finally, there was a significant rise in CD8 levels in the treated group, together with a significant reduction in the CD4/CD8 ratio.

Study by Hirsch et al. [5]

This was a double-blind study versus placebo lasting 1 year, and including 30 children aged between 6 and 16 years, 15 in the treated group and 15 receiving a placebo. The criteria for inclusion were mild to moderate asthma and/or allergic rhinitis caused by mites (8 asthmatics, 8 cases of rhinitis and 14 cases involving both). The criteria used to assess efficacy were the outcome of skin

Table 1. Details of immunotherapy used in the different studies

Tari et al. [4]
Aqueous extract of mites (Neo Abello), 500 STU = 5 BU/ml; 100 BU ≥ 75 mm² of area when prick test in allergics; maintenance: 15 drops of 500 STU 3 times a week; cumulative doses: no data; content of major allergens: no data

Hirsch et al. [5]
Purified whole mite body extract in 50% aqueous glycerol (Allergopharma); maintenance: 7 drops on 3 days per week; 1 drop = 0.535 µg Der p 1; cumulative dose: Der p 1 in 12 months: 570 µg

Passalacqua et al. [6]
Monomeric allergoid DP + DF (Lofarma); maintenance: 2,000 AU twice weekly

Bousquet et al. [7]
Standardized extract of 50% DP + 50% DF (Stallergènes); 1 ml of 100 IR = 8 µg DP + 14 µg DF; maintenance: 20 drops of 300 IR/ml every day for 4 weeks and then 3 days per week for 24 months; cumulative doses: 104,000 IR = 4.2 mg DP + 7.3 mg DF

Mungan et al. [8]
Sublingual immunotherapy
   Standardized extract of 50% DP + 50% DF (Stallergènes); maintenance: 20 drops of
   100 IR/ml every day for 1 month, then 20 drops 2 days a week; cumulative doses:
   11,316 IR in the 1st year; content of major allergens: no data
Subcutaneous immunotherapy
   Calcium phosphate allergenic extract (Stallergènes); maintenance: 0.15–0.75 ml of
   10 IR/ml at 2 weeks' intervals for 3–6 months and then at 4 weeks' intervals; cumulative
   doses: 131 IR; content of major allergens: no data

Guez et al. [9]
Standardized extract of 50% DP + 50% DF (Stallergènes); maintenance: 20 drops of 300 IR/ml every day for 4 weeks and then 3 days per week for 24 months; 1 ml of 300 IR = 4.8 µg DP + 3.7 µg DF; cumulative doses in 24 months: 90,000 IR = 2.2 mg DP + 1.7 mg DF

Pajno et al. [10]
Standardized mite extracts Der p 1 + Der p 2; maintenance dose: 5 drops of 10 BU/ml 3 times a week for 2 years; 10 BU/ml = 4 µg Der p 1 + 2 µg Der p 2; cumulative doses: no data

Bahçeciler et al. [11]
Standardized extract of 50% DP + 50% DF (Stallergènes); maintenance: 20 drops of 100 IR/ml every day for 4 weeks and then 2 days per week for 4 months; 1 ml of 100 IR = 8 µg DP + 14 µg DF; cumulative doses in 6 months: 7,000 IR = 0.56 mg DP + 0.98 mg DF

STU = Standard treatment unit; BU = biological unit; IR = index of reactivity.

Table 2. Determination of allergen exposure in the different studies

	Determination (yes/no)	Method	Modification throughout the study (yes/no)
Tari et al. [4]	yes	guanine	–
Hirsch et al. [5]	yes	ELISA	no
Passalacqua et al. [6]	–	–	–
Bousquet et al. [7]	yes	Acarex test	yes (concentration decreased significantly in both groups)
Mungan et al. [8]	–	–	–
Guez et al. [9]	yes	Acarex test	yes (concentration decreased significantly in active and placebo groups)
Pajno et al. [10]	yes	immunoassay	–
Bahçeciler et al. [11]	–	–	–

– = No data.

Table 3. Tolerance of therapy in the different studies

Tari et al. [4]
In the active group: 3 urticaria, 8 mild asthma, 3 severe asthma, 8 severe nasal symptoms, 6 severe eye symptoms, 4 diarrhea

Hirsch et al. [5]
One severe obstruction in a patient with asthma; 5 local swellings of the tongue (4 treated, 1 on placebo)

Passalacqua et al. [6]
One oral itching in the active group, 1 rhinitis and 1 oral itching in the placebo group

Bousquet et al. [7]
Adverse events in 15 of the 42 patients in the active group and in 14 of the 43 patients on placebo

Mungan et al. [8]
Sublingually active group: 1 buccal pruritis, 1 nausea
Subcutaneous group: 2 local reactions, 1 mild bronchospam

Guez et al. [9]
Two local adverse reactions (mouth itching and burning) in the active group; 1 asthma and 1 episode of rhinosinusitis in the placebo group

Pajno et al. [10]
Tiredness in 4 patients in the active group and in 1 patient on placebo; 1 swelling of mouth and 1 itching of mouth in the active group

Bahçeciler et al. [11]
No local or systemic side effects

tests and the nasal challenge test, and in asthmatics a histamine bronchial challenge test, the assay of specific and total IgE, specific IgG4 levels, symptom and medication scores and a subjective assessment of treatment by patients and physicians.

Results. Eight treated patients and 10 on placebo completed the course of treatment. In 4 treated patients and 3 on placebo, 11 doses were not taken. One treated patient and 1 placebo patient took too many drops at the beginning of the treatment, 1 placebo patient discontinued treatment after 6 weeks and 2 treated patients needed to reduce their maintenance treatment because of the onset of adverse events.

In both groups, a significant improvement could be noted between the beginning and the end of the study, but there was no difference between the treated and placebo groups with regard to skin tests, drug, nasal and bronchial scores, or bronchial challenge test results. In the active group, levels of specific IgE versus mites (*Dermatophagoides pteronyssinus/Dermatophagoides farinae*; DP/DF) were significantly higher than in the placebo group. Treated asthmatic patients saw a greater reduction in symptoms than asthmatics receiving the placebo. However, patients with rhinitis on placebo experienced an improvement in their nasal sensitivity, which was more marked than in the active group (nasal challenge test).

Study by Passalacqua et al. [6]

This was a double-blind, placebo-controlled study of sublingual desensitization in 20 patients, 19 of whom completed the study protocol. The criterion for inclusion was moderate rhinitis-conjunctivitis having progressed for 2 years. There were 9 patients in the placebo group, including 3 smokers, and 10 in the active group, including 4 smokers. Finally, 6 patients also suffered from moderate, intermittent asthma without long-term corticosteroid therapy. The mean ages were 25 years in the active group and 27 years in the placebo group. Efficacy criteria were the daily nasal and conjunctival symptom scores, a conjunctival challenge test (study of early reaction) and a study of intercellular adhesion molecule 1 (ICAM-1) expression, together with the assay of eosinophil cationic protein (ECP) and soluble myeloperoxidase.

Results. In both groups, a seasonal variation in symptoms was observed, which worsened in winter. The treated group experienced fewer allergic symptoms than the placebo group ($p < 0.0002$), with a significant reduction in neutrophil infiltration at the baseline ($p = 0.002$) and during the challenge test ($p = 0.004$), as well as in eosinophil infiltration ($p = 0.001$). The ICAM-1 expression was also reduced. ECP levels diminished significantly in the treated group when compared with the placebo group at the 12th ($p = 0.01$) and

24th month (p = 0.04). Finally, there was a significant reduction in myeloperoxidase levels in the treated group (p = 0.05).

Study by Bousquet et al. [7]

This was a multicenter, double-blind study versus placebo in 85 patients aged from 7 to 42 years, with 42 patients in the active group and 43 in the placebo group; the mean ages in the two groups were 21 and 22 years, respectively, with an even distribution of males and females. The criteria for inclusion were mild to moderate asthma for at least 2 years, excluding patients sensitized to moulds and animal allergens. Associated rhinitis was present in 43% of the active group and 40% of the placebo group. The criteria for efficacy were daily symptom scores with measurement of the peak expiratory flow, the medication score, the outcome of skin tests for mites and other pneumoallergens, a methacholine bronchial challenge test and a quality of life score.

Results. Eighty-five patients were included, 20 were lost to follow-up during the first 6 months (lack of cooperation in the case of 5 in the active group and 4 in the placebo group, lack of efficacy in 1 placebo patient, adverse effects in 5 treated patients and 4 placebo patients). Thus 65 patients completed the study, 32 in the active group and 33 in the placebo group. Although there was no difference between the two groups during the 1st year, at 24 months efficacy based on a global assessment by patients and physicians was better in the treated group than in the placebo group (p = 0.07). Detailed analysis showed that for rhinitis, there were significant differences between the two groups after 11 months (p = 0.02) and 19 months (p = 0.04). The treated group saw a significant reduction in symptoms in comparison with the beginning of treatment (p = 0.006). There was a significant decrease in the medication score after 25 months of treatment. As for asthma, the peak flow rate saw a significant improvement in the treated group in the morning (p = 0.005) and the evening (p = 0.02), with a significant improvement in the forced expiratory volume in 1 s (FEV) and vital capacity in the treated group after 24 months, when compared with the placebo group. Mite concentrations diminished identically and significantly in both groups after 11 and 25 months of treatment. At the end of the treatment period, there was a significant difference between the groups in terms of IgE DP (p = 0.05), IgE DF (p = 0.02) and IgG4 (p = 0.001) regarding DP and DF. There was no difference between the two groups with respect to the bronchial challenge test, but it seems there was an improvement in the treated group while there was no change in the placebo group. As for quality of life, after 25 months of treatment, the highest scores in the treated group concerned mental well-being (p = 0.07), the general perception of well-being (p = 0.01) and physical pain (p = 0.02). There was also a significant difference with respect to social relations in favor of the treated group.

Study by Mungan et al. [8]

This was a study comparing both sublingual and subcutaneous desensitization versus placebo in rhinitis and asthma in 36 patients (7 men and 29 women), with 15 patients in the sublingual group, 10 in the subcutaneous group and 11 in the placebo group. The duration of the study was 1 year. The criteria for inclusion were asthma or rhinitis having progressed for at least 3 years, with a FEV >70%. The criteria for efficacy were the symptom and drug diaries, a reduction in inhaled corticosteroids assessed every 3 months, a methacholine bronchial challenge test, an assay of total IgE, specific IgE and IgG4 and the results of skin tests.

Results. All patients completed the study. There was a significant reduction at 6 months and 1 year in symptom scores concerning rhinitis in the sublingual group ($p < 0.01$) and in the subcutaneous group ($p < 0.05$). As for asthma, the subcutaneous group had a higher symptom score than the sublingual group before the study started ($p = 0.049$). However, there was a significant reduction at 6 months and 1 year in the subcutaneous group ($p < 0.01$) but not in the sublingual group. There was no difference in the placebo group. The sensitivity of skin tests was reduced in the subcutaneous group at 1 year ($p < 0.05$), but there were no changes in the placebo and sublingual groups. There were no changes in any of the groups with respect to levels of specific IgE. As for IgG4, there was a significant increase at 12 months in the sublingual group, and at 6 months and 1 year in the subcutaneous group. Levels in the subcutaneous group were significantly higher ($p < 0.05$) than in the sublingual group at 6 months and 1 year. There were no modifications in any of the groups regarding the results of bronchial challenge tests.

Study by Guez et al. [9]

This study involved 75 patients, 36 in the active group and 36 in the placebo group; 3 patients were excluded because of insufficient data. The mean age of patients was 25 years. The study was conducted double-blind versus placebo for 2 years. The criterion for inclusion was rhinitis with or without asthma. The efficacy criteria were skin tests, a diary kept daily of symptoms and treatments, the assessment of nasal symptoms only, assessment of rhinitis using a visual analog scale by the patient and by the doctor, and assay of specific IgE and specific IgG4 versus mites.

Results. Many more patients withdrew from the study in the placebo group than in the treated group ($p < 0.01$): 21.6 versus 39.5% in the untreated group. Levels of IgE were 18.8 KUI/L in the active group versus 31 in the placebo group, which thus contained more allergic patients. After 24 months of treatment, there was a reduction in the number of patients with scores of 2 and 3 on the Acarex test, with a significant rise in the number of patients scoring 1.

A significant reduction was seen in nasal symptoms in both groups ($p < 0.05$) after 12 months of treatment, and no difference could be seen between the treated and the placebo groups. After 24 months, symptoms had diminished to the same extent in both groups. Nor was there any difference in the global assessments made by doctors. The total medication score fell significantly in both groups between the beginning and the end of the study, but there was no difference between the active and placebo groups. There were no changes to skin test results. IgE levels rose significantly after 12 months of treatment in the active group ($p < 0.05$) but not in the placebo group, and then decreased after 24 months of treatment. There was no difference between the two groups in terms of the evolution of specific IgG4 levels.

Study by Pajno et al. [10]

This was a double-blind study versus placebo conducted in 24 children aged between 8 and 15 years, with 12 patients in the active group and 12 in the placebo group. The study duration was 2 years, after a preinclusion period of 1 year. At the end of the study, 12 patients remained in the active group and 9 in the placebo group. The criteria for inclusion were mild to moderate asthma with $PC_{20} > 2\,mg/ml$ and sensitization solely to mites. The efficacy criteria were the results of skin tests for mites and other pneumoallergens, drug and symptom scores using an analog scale to quantify the severity of symptoms, the assay of specific IgE and IgG4 levels at 12 and 24 months.

Results. There was a significant reduction in the medication score in both groups during the 1st year, with a significant reduction during the 2nd year in the treated group when compared with the placebo group ($p = 0.0066$). Significantly less medication was taken by patients in the treated group ($p = 0.0019$), the greater reduction being seen during the 1st year ($p = 0.0001$). Asthma attacks were seen in both groups during the 1st year of treatment with more attacks in the treated group ($p = 0.02$). There was a significant improvement in both groups during the 2nd year, but this was more marked in the treated group than in patients receiving the placebo ($p = 0.0001$). There was a significant reduction in the number of nighttime awakenings in the treated group during the 2nd year ($p = 0.001$) when compared with the 1st year, and a significant reduction during the 2nd year when compared with the placebo group. Finally, the analog scale had lower scores in the treated group ($p = 0.0001$).

There was no difference with respect to the assays of specific IgE and IgG.

Study by Bahçeciler et al. [11]

This was a double-blind, placebo-controlled study in children with asthma or persistent rhinitis linked to mite allergy. Fifteen children were included: 7 girls and 8 boys with a mean age of 11 years, and they were studied for a period of 6 months.

All patients were monosensitized with a persistence of symptoms despite action to eliminate mites and treatment with inhaled corticosteroids. Patients were included after an 8-week observation period which made it possible to determine the lowest effective dose of budesonide, with the performance of skin tests, lung function tests and a methacholine bronchial challenge test. The efficacy criteria were the medication and symptom scores, global assessment of the patient by the physician, skin tests and total IgE, lung function tests and the methacholine bronchial challenge test.

Results. The results concerned 8 treated patients and 7 on placebo. It was difficult to evaluate the symptom score: there were fewer asthma symptoms in the desensitized group ($p = 0.07$), with an improvement in the daily asthma score which was significant between the beginning and end of desensitization treatment ($p = 0.05$). Patients in the treated group experienced fewer asthma symptoms at the end of treatment, but the result was not significant. As for asthma attacks, the desensitized group had fewer attacks than the placebo group ($p = 0.007$). Regarding the medication score, there was a significant reduction in the intake of β_2-mimetics in the treated group ($p = 0.028$)

At the end of treatment, the mean daily dose of inhaled corticosteroid necessary for the control of asthma was lower in the treated group ($p = 0.06$) but the difference was not significant. An identical trend was seen with respect to the intake of intranasal topical corticosteroids, although within the treated group there was a difference between the beginning and the end of treatment ($p = 0.043$). Within groups, there was a significant difference in the peak expiratory flow in the placebo group between the beginning and end of the study ($p = 0.028$), but no difference in the treated group. The peak flow value in the placebo group was lower than in the active group ($p = 0.049$). There was no difference with respect to bronchial hyperreactivity. Regarding total IgE and skin tests, papule diameters at the end of the study had diminished in the treated group when compared with the placebo group ($p = 0.026$). However, within groups, there were no significant differences, even for total IgE levels.

Discussion

Desensitization against Mites via the Sublingual Route and Therapeutic Efficacy
Is Desensitization via the Sublingual Route More Effective than a Placebo?

A beneficial effect was observed with desensitization to mites via the sublingual route in rhinitis and asthma, with six out of eight studies producing positive results; there was, however, one negative study, where environmental changes masked the effects of desensitization. As for allergic conjunctivitis due to mites, one study was positive and another negative, the former being the best-documented one on conjunctival allergic pathologies, with a reduction in allergic inflammation in the treated group. Thus, overall, the results of the studies were in favor of a beneficial action of specific desensitization via the sublingual route, although we should remember first, the small number of patients studied, and second, the differences (which were sometimes qualitatively and quantitatively minor) in the study parameters between the treated and placebo groups. On the other hand, these studies were extremely rigorous from a methodological point of view; numerous parameters were studied which thus made possible a good analysis of the results and clear validation of the conclusions concerning an improvement in patients following sublingual desensitization.

Is Desensitization via the Sublingual Route More Effective than the Efficient Elimination of Mites?

The sublingual desensitization versus the elimination of mites was not studied, but some data provides an indirect response to this question. In two studies, despite no recommendations having been given to the patients, a significant reduction was seen in the levels of mites in their environment between the beginning and the end of the study. In the study by Bousquet et al. [7], there was nevertheless a greater improvement in rhinitis and asthma in the treated group, while in the study by Guez et al. [9], there was no difference after 2 years between the placebo group and patients treated with sublingual desensitization. However, a larger number of patients discontinued the study in the placebo group than in the treated group.

It, therefore, appeared that satisfactory elimination could significantly improve patients, and also that this elimination was only achieved by patients after several months of follow-up, as they gradually obtained information on it, even if such advice was not given by the investigators. Finally, the association of elimination potentialized the results of the immunotherapy.

Is Sublingual Desensitization against Mites More Effective than Subcutaneous Desensitization?

Only one study considered this very important question, namely that conducted by Mungan et al. [8]. Despite its small population, it appeared that in terms of rhinitis, the two types of allergen administration were equally effective, although this did not apply in the case of asthma, where classic subcutaneous desensitization proved to be superior. However, the authors raised questions as to the doses employed, which differed considerably and may have explained these differences. Thus in allergic rhinitis due to mites, the sublingual route was as effective as the subcutaneous route. In asthma, the effective dose must be established if the results are to equal those obtained with subcutaneous immunotherapy.

Are There Any Criteria Which Predict Better Efficacy with Sublingual Desensitization in Mite Allergy?
Does Age Influence the Results of Desensitization?

Four studies were performed in patients below the age of 18 years [4, 5, 10, 11] and three in adult patients [6, 8, 9], while one included patients both younger and older than 18 years [7]. One study in children was negative as was one in adults. Age, therefore, had no influence on the results of desensitization, although in all cases the patients studied were either children or young adults.

Does the Duration of Treatment Influence Results?

Greater efficacy was achieved with sublingual desensitization when it lasted for more than 1 year, in the knowledge that a major placebo effect was highlighted during the 1st year in two studies [7, 9]. However, there was no objective criterion which limited this treatment to 2 years; on the contrary, several studies produced positive results after 6 months of treatment.

Does the Type and Concentration of the Products Used
Affect the Results?

It is very difficult to compare results between different studies, because the treatment units and products employed were not the same. Despite this, it seems that higher doses were more effective, without any relationship being seen between dosage and adverse effects.

Disadvantages and Adverse Effects of Sublingual Desensitization in Mite Allergy
Were There Any Major Adverse Effects?

Except for one study [4] which reported 32 adverse events (!!), all studies emphasized the benignity of the rare adverse effects observed. The reputed safety of this desensitization method thus seems to be true, particularly if the results of all published studies on sublingual desensitization were grouped together, regardless of the allergen employed [12, 13].

Was Patient Compliance with the Treatment Satisfactory?

In the study by Hirsch et al. [5], 9 out of 30 patients made mistakes with their dosage at the beginning of the treatment. In the study of Bousquet et al. [7], there was a high rate of withdrawal at the beginning of the study (20 patients out of 85). In the study of Guez et al. [9], numerous withdrawals were also seen, particularly in the placebo group (39.5 vs. 21.68%), with 25 patients in the treated group and 14 patients in the placebo group completing the study (initially, there were 36 patients in each group). It, therefore, appears that compliance with the treatment was easier for children than for adults.

Questions Not Answered Concerning Sublingual Desensitization in Mite Allergy

Does sublingual desensitization preclude subsequent sensitizations? Are the benefits of desensitization sustained for a long time after its discontinuation? Is a maximum duration of 24 months justified by objective arguments? As yet, no study has provided an answer to these questions concerning sublingual desensitization in mite allergy.

Conclusion

Desensitization to mites via the sublingual route offers a second opportunity [3] for specific immunotherapy, which has widely proved its benefit via the subcutaneous route, but often at the price of serious adverse effects. In this respect, the sublingual route is indeed a treatment which only causes minor adverse effects. So far, fewer studies have been published concerning its efficacy than that of subcutaneous desensitization, but these studies are much more rigorous from a methodological point of view. The findings of these studies seem to confirm the efficacy of sublingual desensitization in mite allergy, when it is associated with the efficient elimination of mites in the environment [14, 15]. However, assessments of these results differ, depending on the analytical criteria applied. Thus, in Europe, allergologists seem to be in favor of prescribing this sublingual method of desensitization first in patients allergic to mites, while in the United States, sublingual desensitization only constitutes a useful alternative when subcutaneous desensitization is not possible [16]. It is, therefore, necessary to do studies, but in much larger populations of patients, so that we can definitively confirm the efficacy of sublingual desensitization in patients allergic to mites.

Acknowledgments

We thank Dr. Hervé Masson for helpful discussions and Dr. Jocelyne Gasteau for her help with the translation of this manuscript.

References

1   Frew AJ, White PJ, Smith HE: Sublingual immunotherapy. J Allergy Clin Immunol 1999;104/2: 267–270.
2   de Blay F, Casel S, Spirlet F, Pauli G: Eviction des allergènes: intérêts et limites. Rev Fr Allergol Immunol Clin 2000;40:367–371.
3   Bousquet J, Lockey RF, Malling HJ: WHO position paper. Allergen immunotherapy: Therapeutic vaccines for allergic diseases. Allergy 1998;53(suppl):1–42.
4   Tari MG, Mancino M, Monti G: Efficacy of sublingual immunotherapy in patients with rhinitis and asthma due to house dust mite. A double-blind study. Allergol Immunopathol 1990;18:277–284.
5   Hirsch TH, Sähn M, Leupold W: Double-blind placebo-controlled study of sublingual immunotherapy with house dust mite extract (D.pt.) in children. Pediatr Allergy Immunol 1997;8:21–27.
6   Passalacqua G, Albano M, Fregonese L, Riccio A, Pronzato C, Mela GS, Canonica GW: Randomised controlled trial of local allergoid immunotherapy on allergic inflammation in mite-induced rhinoconjunctivitis. Lancet 1998;351:629–632.
7   Bousquet J, Scheinmann P, Guinnepain MT, Perrin-Fayolle M, Sauvaget J, Tonnel AB, Pauli G, Caillaud D, Dubost R, Leynadier F, Vervloet D, Herman D, Galvain S, André C: Sublingual-swallow immunotherapy (SLIT) in patients with asthma due to house-dust mites: A double-blind, placebo-controlled study. Allergy 1999;55:249–260.
8   Mungan D, Misirligil Z, Gürbüz L: Comparison of the efficacy of subcutaneous and sublingual immunotherapy in mite-sensitive patients with rhinitis and asthma. A placebo controlled study. Ann Allergy Asthma Immunol 1999;82:485–490.
9   Guez S, Vatrinet C, Fadel R, André C: House-dust-mite sublingual-swallow immunotherapy (SLIT) in perennial rhinitis: A double-blind, placebo-controlled study. Allergy 2000;55:369–375.
10 Pajno GB, Morabito L, Barberio G, Parmiani S: Clinical and immunologic effects of long-term sublingual immunotherapy in asthmatic children sensitized to mites: A double-blind, placebo-controlled study. Allergy 2000;55:842–849.
11 Bahçeciler NN, Isik U, Barlan IB, Basaran MM: Efficacy of sublingual immunotherapy in children with asthma and rhinitis: A double-blind, placebo-controlled study. Pediatr Pulmonol 2001;32:49–55.
12 André C, Vatrinet C, Galvain S, Carat F, Sicard H: Safety of sublingual-swallow immunotherapy in children and adults. Int Arch Allergy Immunol 2000;121:229–234.
13 Lombardi C, Gargioni S, Melchiorre A, Tiri A, Falagiani P, Canonica GW, Pasalacqua G: Safety of sublingual immunotherapy with monomeric allergoid in adults: Multicenter post-marketing surveillance study. Allergy 2001;56:989–992.
14 Rakoski J, Wessner D: A short assessment of sublingual immunotherapy. Int Arch Allergy Immunol 2001;126:185–187.
15 Passalacqua G, Canonica GW: Allergen-specific sublingual immunotherapy for respiratory allergy. BioDrugs 2001;15:509–519.
16 Frew AJ, Smith HE: Sublingual immunotherapy. J Allergy Clin Immunol 2001;107:441–444.

Stéphane Guez, MD, Unité des Maladies Allergiques,
Service de Médecine Interne 3.3, Hôpital Pellegrin-Tripode,
CHU, F–33076 Bordeaux Cedex (France)
Tel. +33 556795541, Fax +33 556794804, E-Mail stephane.guez@chu-bordeaux.fr

Markert UR, Elsner P (eds): Local Immunotherapy in Allergy.
Chem Immunol Allergy. Basel, Karger, 2003, vol 82, pp 77–88

······················

Efficacy of Sublingual Immunotherapy in Asthma and Eczema

G.B. Pajno[a], *D.G. Peroni*[b], *G. Barberio*[a], *A.L. Boner*[b]

[a] Department of Paediatrics, University of Messina, Messina, and
[b] Department of Paediatrics, University of Verona, Verona, Italy

---

Key Words

Allergy · Asthma · Eczema · Immunotherapy · Rhinitis

Abstract

Sublingual immunotherapy (SLIT) is the local route of administration of allergen extracts investigated in several controlled clinical trials. In a number of countries, particularly Italy, France and Spain, this has become common in office practice. At variance with subcutaneous immunotherapy, the knowledge of mechanisms of action of SLIT is still at the beginning: some studies, in animal models, provided interesting information: the dendritic cells of oral mucosa act as efficient antigen-presenting cells and produce IL-12, which directs the immune response towards a Th1 profile away from IgE-Th2 profile. Its clinical efficacy (improvement of symptoms and reduction of drug intake) for both asthma and rhinitis has been assessed in detail for the most common allergens: house dust mites, grass pollen, *Parietaria*, birch pollen and olive tree. SLIT requires further evaluation concerning the treatment of the extrinsic form of atopic dermatitis. The induction of immunologic tolerance rather than immunoreactivity should be worth pursuing due to the immunologic pathway involved in the pathophysiology of atopic dermatitis. The safety profile of SLIT, derived from the clinical trials and postmarketing surveillance studies, turned out to be satisfactory in adults and children. SLIT represents an important step towards an efficacious and safe treatment of patients with allergic respiratory diseases; nevertheless, further studies are necessary to establish it as a viable alternative to subcutaneous immunotherapy.

Introduction

The interest in the local routes of administration for immunotherapy (IT) has rapidly increased, and a large number of clinical trials have been published within the last few years. These routes have the primary aim of minimizing the risk of adverse events and of improving patients' acceptance of treatment [1]. In a number of countries, particularly Italy, France and Spain this has become common in office practice, and there is also an increasing body of evidence from academic studies to support the practice of local IT [1]. The rationale for the use of local IT derives from the observation that activated T lymphocytes are able to migrate from one mucosal site to another [2–4]. Furthermore, asthmatic patients exhibit an 'airway-like' inflammation of various mucosal sites (like gut mucosa or minor salivary glands), suggesting that the whole mucosal system is involved as a cause or as a consequence in asthma [5].

An intriguing question concerns the immune response elicited by allergen extracts at the mucosal surface. Some studies, in animal models, provided interesting information: the dendritic cells of oral mucosa act as efficient antigen-presenting cells and produce IL-12, which directs the immune response towards a Th1 profile away from pro-IgE-Th2 profile [6–8].

In contrast to animal models, the immunologic response to sublingual immunotherapy (SLIT) in humans has been difficult to demonstrate. Specific IgE suppression, specific IgG production or changes in the T cell-cytokine profile seem to be little affected by SLIT [9–13].

After the administration of the ^{123}I-radiolabeled allergen (Par j 1) in adult volunteers sequential scintiscanning did not show direct absorption of the allergen through the mucosa and plasma radioactivity increased only after the allergen was swallowed [14]. Moreover, the allergen was retained for long time (up to 40 h) in the oral mucosa. These data showed that there is no risk of rapid absorption of the allergen through the oral mucosa, the antigens being retained locally. It is very likely that antigens are processed in the local oral immune system [15].

Efficacy of SLIT in Asthma

In the 1998 EAACI position paper 6 studies using the sublingual route were identified [1]. The authors concluded that SLIT had been shown to be efficacious in patients with rhinitis, but insufficient information was available to draw any conclusions for its use in asthma.

Since 1998, a number of further studies have been published. Nowadays we can rely on 19 double-blind placebo-controlled studies, performed with adequate methods and samples as summarized in table 1 [10, 12, 16–32]. Six of these studies were performed in pediatric patients [16–21]. Almost all the studies confirmed the effectiveness of SLIT with grass extracts. Mite, birch and *Parietaria* extracts showed apparent favorable results in terms of symptom improvement and/or reduction of the intake of rescue medications. But the effects were inconsistent: some studies showed no influence on asthma and others no difference in drug consumption (table 1). In two studies [17, 22] both conducted with mite extracts, SLIT efficacy was poor: a trend toward clinical improvement was seen in the active groups but it did not reach the statistical significance.

In patients allergic to mites, the duration of the treatment seems to be crucial: a long-lasting treatment with a high dose of allergen may provide positive results [20] (fig. 1). It is important to notice that SLIT could exert its effects not only on rhinitis but also on asthma symptoms. The results from recent studies showed that there is a clear-cut reduction of the clinical symptom score [20, 23, 24], the days with asthma symptoms [25], as well as the use of β_2-agonists [21, 25], and the use of systemic steroids [32].

There is very limited information about the comparative efficacy of the different routes (i.e. sublingual or subcutaneous) of administration of allergens in IT. One single double-blind double-dummy study showed that SLIT had a clinical efficacy similar to that of subcutaneous IT (SIT) for symptom reduction and the need of drugs [33]. On the other hand, objective parameters (total specific IgG, specific IgG4, skin reactivity) changed only in patients treated with active injection therapy. SLIT was in any case better accepted and tolerated by patients [33]. Another placebo-controlled, parallel-group, single-blind study was performed in adult patients sensitive to mites [34]. SIT for both rhinitis and asthma was clinically effective. Patients treated with SLIT had decreased rhinitis symptoms (p < 0.01), but no change in asthma scores [34].

The recent study by Wilson et al. [35], published so far in abstract form, compared clinical and laboratory data from two IT trials performed concurrently during one grass pollen season in patients with moderate/severe hay fever. Two double-blind placebo-controlled studies one employing injection and the other high-dose (50 times subcutaneous dose) SLIT administration of allergen were performed in parallel in a single center. SLIT had a clinical efficacy around 65% of the efficacy of SIT. Reduction in allergen sensitivity, both early and late, and increases in protective IgG4 were significantly greater following SIT [35].

There are no studies comparing the efficacy of SLIT and drugs. Such trials would be of interest to answer the question of how IT compares with pharmacotherapy. It is important, however, to reinforce the concept that both therapies are complementary and that very likely the combination of both strategies will provide the patient with better options for both symptom control and possibly for modification of the natural history of the disease [36].

Concerning the dose of SLIT, the cumulative up-dosing of allergen used in SLIT studies has been between 3.25 and 375 times the dose of allergen given

Table 1. Double-blind placebo-controlled sublingual IT studies

Author, year	Patients' age range	Allergen	Duration months	Cumulative dose	Patients IT	Patients Placebo	Disease	Results	Drug consumption
Tari et al., 1990 [16]	5–12	mites	12–18	720 BU	30	28	R/A	R = p < 0.001 A = p < 0.001	NS
Sabbah et al., 1994 [28]	13–51	grass	4	4,500 IR	29	29	R	R < 0.05	NS p < 0.05
Feliziani et al., 1995 [27]	14–48	grass	3.5	720 BU	18	16	R/A	R = p < 0.01 A = p = 0.026	R = p = 0.002 A = p < 0.05
Troise et al., 1995 [12]	17–60	Parietaria	10	105 BU (Par 1 6.3)	15	16	R	p < 0.02	p < 0.05
Hirsh et al., 1997 [17]	6–16	mites	12	570 µg Der p 1	15	15	R/A	R = NS A ≤ 0.05	NR
Passalacqua et al., 1998 [31]	15–46	mites	24	10,000 AU	10	10	R/A	p = 0.05	NR
Vourdas et al., 1998 [18]	7–17	olive	24	8.1 mg Ole e 1	33	31	R/A	R < 0.05 A < 0.04	NR
Clavel et al., 1998 [32]	8–55	grass	6	40,700 IR 2.6 mg Phl p 5	62	58	R/A	R = NS A = p < 0.02	R = p < 0.05 A = p < 0.01
Horak et al., 1998 [29]	18–48	birch	4	9,250 STU	21	20	R	R = NS	NR
Nelson et al., 1993 [10]	18–74	cat	3–4	4,500,000 AU	20	21	R	NS	NR
Hordijk et al., 1998 [26]	18–45	grass	10	798,000 BU	30	27	R	P < 0.03	NS
Bousquet et al., 1999 [23]	15–37	mites	25	104,000 IR 4.2 mg Der p 1, 7.3 mg Der f 1	32	33	R/A	R < 0.05 A = NS	NS
Passalacqua et al., 1999 [30]	15–42	Parietaria	5	256 BU 16 µg Par j 1	14	10	R/A	R = NS A = NS	NR

Study	Age	Allergen	Duration	Dose	Treated	Control	R/A	Rhinitis	Asthma/other
Pradalier et al., 1999 [25]	7–58	grass	4	11,000 IR 0.935 mg Phl p 5	60	59	R/A	R = NS A < 0.02	NS
La Rosa et al., 1999 [19]	6–14	*Parietaria*	24	150,000 IR 52.3 µg Par j 1	16	17	R	= 0.02	NS
Purello-D'Ambrosio et al., 1999 [24]	14–50	*Parietaria*	9	200 BU 12.7 µg Par j 1	14	16	R/A	> 0.05	NS
Pajno et al., 2000 [20]	8–15	mites	24	7,500 BU 0.8 mg Der p 1, 0.4 mg Der p 2	12	12	A	p = 0.0001	p = 0.0001
Guez et al., 2000 [22]	6–51	mites	24	90,000 IR 2.2 mg Der p 1, 1.7 mg Der f 2	25	14	R	NS	NS
Caffarelli 2000 [21]	4–14	grass	3	37,250 AU	24	20	R/A	R = NS A = p < 0.05	NS

NS = Not significant; NR = not reported; R = rhinitis; A = asthma.

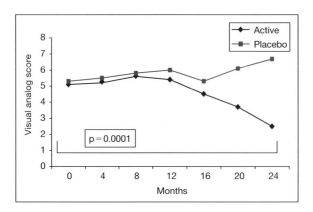

Fig. 1. Visual analog score on overall asthma symptoms for active SLIT and placebo groups. Data points represent average 4-month visual analog scores [20].

to patients for conventional SIT [19, 20]. The use of a high dose of SLIT is probably the key for the successful treatment of the patients together with the long-term duration of therapy [37].

Efficacy of SLIT in Eczema

Atopic dermatitis (AD) is a chronic, relapsing, pruritic, and inflammatory skin disease that frequently predates the development of allergic rhinitis and asthma [38].

Immunologic triggers of AD are food allergens [39], bacteria, fungi and inhalant allergens [40, 41].

Different clinical studies suggest that inhalation or contact with aeroallergens (especially house dust mites) may exacerbate AD [reviewed in 38]. Nevertheless, there are very few studies regarding the treatment of AD.

A double-blind controlled trial of hyposensitization with tyrosine-adsorbed *Dermatophagoides pteronyssinus* (Dpt) vaccine in 24 children with atopic eczema and immediate hypersensitivity to Dpt failed to demonstrate superiority over placebo after a standard 8 months of treatment [42]. Twenty-four adults with AD and hypersensitivity to Dpt were treated in another double-blind, placebo-controlled trial by intradermal injections of complexes containing autologous specific antibodies and mite allergens [43]. After 4 months, placebo-treated patients started receiving active treatment. All patients were treated for a full year. Symptoms of AD subsided within a few weeks after starting therapy, with a significant reduction after 4 months in treated patients only. After 1 year,

Table 2. Role of Th2/Th1 cytokines in AD [64]

	Uninvolved skin	Acute skin	Chronic skin
Cell type			
T cells	+	+++	++
Eosinophils	0	+	+++
Macrophages	0	++	+++
Cytokine gene expression			
IL-4, IL-13	+	++++	+++
IL-5	0	++	+++
IFN-γ	0	0	++
IL-12	0	0	++
IL-16	+	+++	++
GM-CSF	0	+	++

82% of the patients exhibited a mean improvement of 83%, associated with a reduction of Dpt-specific IgG antibodies [43].

Other studies have been performed in canine AD with variable results from a poor to a good response [44–46]. Better results were obtained when specific IT was started early at the onset of disease [44]. A task force on canine AD advocated that allergen-specific IT may be included in the treatment of canine AD because of its potential advantages and limited disadvantages compared to other forms of therapy [47]. It seems that there is more experience with this practice in dogs than in humans.

Observational studies with SLIT in humans with AD claimed favorable results [48–50]. However, these studies do not allow definitive conclusions and so far the amount and quality of information regarding this issue are not sufficient to formulate any formal recommendation if not that of an urgent need of properly double-blind, placebo-controlled studies.

Furthermore, the immunologic pathway involved in the pathophysiology of AD is complex (table 2). It presents a degree of complexity which has not been appreciated with allergic rhinitis and asthma. In AD both Th1 and Th2 T cell products play a role in chronic inflammation, which is maintained by both IL-5 (Th2) and IFN-γ (Th1) [51]. In addition recent studies have demonstrated different cytokine expressions in acute (predominantly IL-16) and in chronic (mainly IL-12 and GM-CSF) lesions [52, 53].

The increased expression of IL-12 in chronic AD skin lesions is of interest since this cytokine plays a key role in the Th1 cell development. For these reasons the induction of Th1 response by allergen-specific IT [54] may be theoretically

Table 3. SLIT: characteristics of reported side effects [57]

Side effects	Episodes	Patients%	Grade	Onset
Conjunctival itching	1	0.37	mild	<30 min
Abdominal pain	1	0.37	mild	<30 min
Rhinitis	5	1.9	mild	<30 min
Urticaria	1	0.37	moderate	<30 min
Total	8	3		

harmful to some patients suffering from eczema. For AD the induction of immunologic tolerance rather than immunoreactivity should be worth pursuing.

Safety of SLIT

In childhood the main concern about the use of SLIT is the safety aspect [55–58], and, at present, few data are available on large numbers of treated patients. A review article of eight placebo-controlled trials in children with allergic rhinitis and/or asthma disclosed adverse events in 48% of the 103 subjects receiving the active treatment, but no severe reaction was observed [59]. All the surveys on SLIT disclosed an incidence of mild to moderate unwanted effects, which is lower than that reported for SIT and no life-threatening side effects [57, 60]. Oral/sublingual itching and local gastrointestinal symptoms (especially abdominal pain) are the most common adverse events in all studies and are usually classified as local side effects because the allergens were earlier kept in the mouth for at least 2 min and then swallowed. Systemic side effects (rhinitis, urticaria, wheezing) were also reported; however, no life-threatening events were reported by patients (table 3).

In a recent personal evaluation of side effects related to SLIT in 354 children suffering from allergic asthma and followed for at least 39 months no adverse event was observed in 90.4% of the children [61]. We observed 0.155 mild to moderate reactions per 1,000 administrations. In 15 episodes only dosage adjustment was required. In 5 children IT was stopped as a precaution. No anaphylactic reaction or multiple-organ life-threatening event occurred [61].

Conclusions

The therapy of respiratory allergy should be based on allergen avoidance, pharmacological treatment and, when indicated, IT [37]. SLIT represents a significant advantage in terms of patient acceptability and reduction of medical supervision, but several aspects need to be better studied before its broad application in allergic children [62]. First, SLIT appears to be less effective than SIT [35] and second, a modification of the cellular response to allergen has not yet been demonstrated after SLIT [62].

We need long-term prospective studies comparing SLIT with SIT, before abandoning a practice which has been shown to be effective [63] in favor of a safe practice which has not yet been completely demonstrated to be efficacious, particularly in asthmatic patients. Further evaluations of SLIT are necessary concerning the treatment of the extrinsic form of AD.

The balance sheet for SLIT is improving; SLIT represents an important step towards an adequate treatment of patients with allergic respiratory diseases; nevertheless, the safety of an alternative therapy is only a real advantage if it is not counterbalanced by a loss of efficacy.

Appendix

Standardization of Extracts

Index of reactivity (IR) units: The in-house reference extract (called 100 IR) is defined as the concentration eliciting a wheal with a mean diameter of 7 mm in 30 skin-tested patients with allergies.

Biologically standardized unit (BU) extracts are quantified in mass units. 100 BU/ml is the concentration of allergen able to elicit a mean wheal of 75 mm^2 when prick-tested in 30 allergic subjects.

Allergic unit (AU) is a biologic unit originally established to titrate products for intranasal IT and is defined as 1/40 of the mean provocative dose by specific nasal challenge in a significant number of allergic volunteers.

References

1   Malling HJ, Abreu-Nogueira J, Alvarez-Cuesta E, et al: Local immunotherapy (position paper). Allergy 1998;53:933–944.
2   Mestecky J: The common mucosal immune system and current strategies for induction of immune responses in external secretions. J Clin Immunol 1987;4:265–276.
3   Bienenstock J, Befus D, McDermott S, et al: Regulation of lymphoblast traffic and localization in mucosal tissue, with emphasis on IgA. Fed Proc 1983;42:3213–3217.
4   Mackay CR, Marston WL, Dusdler L: Naïve and memory T cells show distinct pathways of lymphocyte recirculation. J Exp Med 1990;171:801–817.
5   Wallaert B, Lamblin C, Tsicopoulos A, et al: Asthma –More than a bronchial disease? ACI Int 2000;12:161–165.
6   Hasseus B, Dahlgren V, Bergenholtz G, Jontell M: Antigen presenting capacity of Langerhans cells from rat oral epithelium. J Oral Pathol Med 1995;24:56–60.
7   Van Wilsem EJ, Van Hoogstraatn IM, Breve J, et al: Dendritic cells of the oral mucosa and the induction of oral tolerance. Immunology 1994;83:128–132.

8 Macatinia SE, Hosken NA, Litton M, et al: Dendritic cells produce IL-12 and direct the development of Th1 cells form naïve CD4+ T cells. J Exp Med 1993;177:1199–1204.

9 Tari MG, Mancino M, Madonna F, et al: Immunologic evaluation of 24 month course of sublingual immunotherapy. Allergol Immunopathol 1994;22:209–216.

10 Nelson HS, Hoppenheimer J, Vatsia GA, Buchmeier A: A double-blind placebo-controlled evaluation of sublingual immunotherapy with standardized cat extract. J Allergy Clin Immunol 1993;92:229–236.

11 Casanovas M, Guerra F, Moreno C, et al: Double-blind placebo-controlled clinical trial of preseasonal immunotherapy with allergenic extracts of *Olea europea* pollen administered sublingually. J Invest Allergol Clin Immunol 1994;4:305–314.

12 Troise C, Voltolini S, Canessa A, et al: Sublingual immunotherapy in Parietaria pollen-induced rhinitis: A double-blind study. J Invest Allergol Clin Immunol 1995;5:25–30.

13 Fanta C, Bohle B, Hirt W, et al: Systemic immunological changes induced by administration of grass pollen allergens via the oral mucosa during sublingual immunotherapy. Int Arch Allergy Appl Immunol 1999;120:218–224.

14 Bagnasco M, Mariani G, Passalacqua G, et al: Absorption and distribution kinetics of the major *Parietaria judaica* allergen (Par j 1) administered by noninjectable routes in healthy human beings. J Allergy Clin Immunol 1997;100:122–129.

15 Bagnasco M, Passalacqua G, Villa G, et al: Pharmacokinetics of an allergen and a monomeric allergoid for oromucosal immunotherapy in allergic volunteers. Clin Exp Allergy 2001;31:54–60.

16 Tari MG, Mancino M, Monti G: Efficacy of sublingual immunotherapy in patients with rhinitis and asthma due to house dust mite. A double-blind study. Allergol Immunopathol 1990;18:277–284.

17 Hirsch T, Sahm M, Leupold W: Double-blind placebo controlled study of sublingual immunotherapy with house dust mite extracts in children. Pediatr Allergy Immunol 1997;8:21–27.

18 Vourdas D, Syrigou E, Potamianou P, et al: Double-blind placebo controlled evaluation of sublingual immunotherapy with a standardized olive tree pollen extract in pediatric patients with allergic rhinoconjunctivitis and mild asthma due to olive tree pollen sensitization. Allergy 1998;53:662–671.

19 La Rosa M, Ranno C, André C, et al: Double-blind placebo controlled evaluation of sublingual swallow immunotherapy with standardized *Parietaria judaica* extract in children with allergic rhinoconjunctivitis. J Allergy Clin Immunol 1999;104:425–432.

20 Pajno GB, Morabito L, Barberio G, Parmiani S: Clinical and immunological effects of long-term sublingual immunotherapy in asthmatic children sensitized to mite: A double-blind study. Allergy 2000;55:842–849.

21 Caffarelli C: Preseasonal local allergoid immunotherapy to grass pollen in children: A double-blind, placebo-controlled randomized trial. Allergy 2000;55:1–6.

22 Guez S, Vatrinet C, Fadel R, André C: House dust mite sublingual swallow immunotherapy in perennial rhinitis: A double-blind placebo-controlled study. Allergy 2000;55:369–375.

23 Bousquet J, Scheinman P, Guinnepain MT, et al: Sublingual swallow immunotherapy (SLIT) in patients with asthma due to house dust mites: A double-blind placebo-controlled study. Allergy 1999;54:249–260.

24 Purello-D'Ambrosio F, Gangemi S, Isola S, et al: Sublingual immunotherapy: A double-blind placebo-controlled trial with *Parietaria judaica* extract standardized in mass units in patients with rhinoconjunctivitis, asthma or both. Allergy 1999;54:968–973.

25 Pradalier A, Basset D, Claudel A, et al: Sublingual swallow immunotherapy (SLIT) with a standardized five grass pollen extract (drops and sublingual tablets) versus placebo in seasonal rhinitis. Allergy 1999;54:819–828.

26 Hordijk GJ, Antvelink JB, Luwema RA: Sublingual immunotherapy with a standardized grass pollen extract; a double-blind placebo-controlled study. Allergol Immunopathol 1998;26:234–240.

27 Feliziani V, Lattuada G, Parmiani S, et al: Safety and efficacy of sublingual rush immunotherapy with grass allergen extracts. A double blind study. Allergol Immunopathol 1995;23:224–230.

28 Sabbah A, Hassoun S, Le Sellin J, et al: A double-blind, placebo-controlled trial by the sublingual route of immunotherapy with a standardized grass pollen extract. Allergy 1994;49:309–313.

29 Horak F, Stubne P, Berger UE, et al: Immunotherapy with sublingual birch pollen extract. A short-term double blind placebo study. Invest Allergol Clin Immunol 1998;8:165–171.

30   Passalacqua G, Albano M, Riccio A, et al: Clinical and immunologic effects of a rush sublingual immunotherapy to Parietaria species: A double-blind, placebo-controlled trial. J Allergy Clin Immunol 1999;104:964–968.

31   Passalacqua G, Albano M, Fregonese L, et al: Randomized controlled trial of local allergoid immunotherapy on allergic inflammation in mite-induced rhinoconjunctivitis. Lancet 1998;351:629–632.

32   Clavel R, Bousquet J, André C: Clinical efficacy of sublingual swallow immunotherapy: A double-blind placebo controlled trial of a standardized five grass pollen extract in rhinitis. Allergy 1998; 53:493–498.

33   Quirino T, Iemali E, Siciliani E, Parmiani S: Sublingual vs injective immunotherapy in grass pollen allergic patients: A double-blind double-dummy study. Clin Exp Allergy 1996;26:1253–1261.

34   Mungan D, Misirligil Z, Gurbuz L: Comparison of the efficacy of subcutaneous and sublingual immunotherapy in mite-sensitive patients with rhinitis and asthma – A placebo controlled study. Ann Allergy Asthma Immunol 1999;82:485–490.

35   Wilson DR, Walker SM, Torres Lima M, Durham SR: Comparison between injection and sublingual immunotherapy for hay fever: Diary scores, skin responsiveness and serum antibodies. J Allergy Clin Immunol 2002;109:S170.

36   Moller C, Dreborg S, Ferdousi HA, et al: Pollen immunotherapy reduces the development of asthma in children with seasonal rhinoconjunctivitis (the PAT-study). J Allergy Clin Immunol 2002;109:251–256.

37   Bousquet J, Khaltaev N, Van Cauwenberge P: Rhinitis and its impact on asthma (ARIA). WHO position paper. J Allergy Clin Immunol 2001;108(suppl 5):240–247.

38   Leung DYM: Atopic dermatitis: New insight and opportunities for therapeutic intervention. J Allergy Clin Immunol 2000;105:860–872.

39   Eingenmann PA, Sicherer SH, Borkowski TA, et al: Prevalence of IgE-mediated food allergy among children with atopic dermatitis. Pediatrics 1998;101/3:E8.

40   Lever R, Hadley K, Downey D, et al: Staphylococcal colonization in atopic dermatitis and the effect of topical mupirocin therapy. Br J Dermatol 1988;119:189–198.

41   Scalabrin DM, Bavbek S, Perzanowski MS, et al: Use of specific IgE in assessing the relevance of fungal and dust mite allergens to atopic dermatitis: A comparison with asthmatic and nonasthmatic control subjects. J Allergy Clin Immunol 1999;104:1273–1279.

42   Glover MT, Atherton DJ: A double-blind controlled trial of hyposensitization to *Dermatophagoides pteronyssinus* in children with atopic eczema. Clin Exp Allergy 1992;22:440–446.

43   Leroy BP, Boden G, Lachapelle JM, et al: A novel therapy for atopic dermatitis with allergen-antibody complexes: A double-blind placebo-controlled study. J Am Acad Dermatol 1993;28: 232–239.

44   Nuttall TJ, Thoday KL, van den Broek AH, et al: Retrospective survey of allergen immunotherapy in canine atopy. Vet Rec 1998;143:139–142.

45   Park S, Ohya F, Yamashita K, et al: Comparison of response to immunotherapy by intradermal skin test and antigen-specific IgE in canine atopy. J Vet Med Sci 2000;62:983–988.

46   Mueller RS, Bettenay SV: Evaluation of the safety of an abbreviated course of injections of allergen extracts for the treatment of dogs with atopic dermatitis. Am J Vet Res 2001;62:307–310.

47   Griffin CE, Hillier A: The ACVD task force on canine atopic dermatitis: Allergen-specific immunotherapy. Vet Immunol Immunopathol 2001;81:363–383.

48   Galli E, Chini L, Nardi S: Use of oral hyposensitization therapy to *Dermatophagoides pteronyssinus* in children with atopic dermatitis. Allergol Immunopathol 1994;22:18–22.

49   Mastrandrea F, Serio G, Minelli M: Specific sublingual immunotherapy in atopic dermatitis. Results of a 6-year follow-up of 35 consecutive patients. Allergol Immunopathol 2000;28:54–62.

50   Pacor ML, Biasi D, Maleknia T: The efficacy of long-term specific immunotherapy for *Dermatophagoides pteronyssinus* in patients with atopic dermatitis. Recenti Prog Med 1994;85: 273–277.

51   Hamid Q, Boguniewicz M, Leung DYM: Differential cytokine gene expression in acute vs chronic atopic dermatitis. J Clin Invest 1994;94:870–876.

52   Hamid Q, Naseer T, Minshall EM, et al: In vivo expression of interleukin-12 and interleukin-13 in atopic dermatitis. J Allergy Clin Immunol 1996;98:225–231.

53   Laberge S, Ghaffar O, Boguniewicz M, et al: Association of increased CD4+ T-cell infiltration with increased IL-16 gene expression in atopic dermatitis. J Allergy Clin Immunol 1998;102: 645–650.
54   Durham SR, Till SJ: Immunologic changes associated with allergen immunotherapy. J Allergy Clin Immunol 1998;102:157–164.
55   Malling HJ, Abreu-Noguiera J, Alvarez-Cuesta E, et al: EAACI/ESPACI position paper: Local immunotherapy. Allergy 1998;53:933–944.
56   Tari MG, Mancino M, Monti G: Efficacy of sublingual immunotherapy in patients with rhinitis and asthma due to house dust mite. A double-blind study. Allergol Immunopathol (Madr) 1990; 18:277–284.
57   Di Rienzo V, Pagani A, Parmiani S, et al: Post-marketing surveillance study on the safety of sublingual immunotherapy in pediatric patients. Allergy 1999;54:1110–1113.
58   Brown JL, Frew AJ: The efficacy of oromucosal immunotherapy in respiratory allergy. Clin Exp Allergy 2001;31:8–10.
59   André C, Vatrinet C, Galvain S, et al: Safety of sublingual-swallow immunotherapy in children and adults. Int Arch Allergy Immunol 2000;121:229–234.
60   Lombardi C, Gargioni S, Melchiorre A, et al: Safety of sublingual immunotherapy with monomeric allergoid in adults: Multicentre post-marketing surveillance study. Allergy 2001;56: 989–992.
61   Pajno GB, Peroni DG, Boner AL: Safety of sublingual immunotherapy in asthmatic children. Paediatric Drugs, submitted.
62   Frew AJ: Sublingual immunotherapy. J Allergy Clin Immunol 2001;107:441–444.
63   Ross RN, Nelson HS, Finegold I: Effectiveness of specific immunotherapy in the treatment of asthma: A meta-analysis of prospective, randomised, double-blind, placebo-controlled studies. Clin Ther 2000;22:329–341.
64   Charlesworth EN: AAAAI 58th Annual Meeting – Postgraduate Syllabus, New York, 2002, pp 191–199.

Dr. Giovanni Battista Pajno
Divisione Pediatria 2°, Policlinico Universitario,
Via Consolare Valeria – Gazzi, I-98124 Messina (Italy)
Tel. +39 090 2213162, Fax +39 090 2212143, E-Mail Giovanni.Pajno@unime.it

Markert UR, Elsner P (eds): Local Immunotherapy in Allergy.
Chem Immunol Allergy. Basel, Karger, 2003, vol 82, pp 89–98

....

Nasal Application of Immunotherapy

E. Ascione, A. De Lucia, M. Imperiali, A. Varricchio, G. Motta

ENT Institute, Second University of Naples, Naples, Italy

Key Words

Immunotherapy · Allergic rhinitis · Iposensitization · Allergen specific · Prophylaxis

Abstract

Background: In patients with allergic rhinitis local nasal immunotherapy (LNIT) appears to offer considerable advantages over other hyposensitization methods. The aim of our study was to obtain further confirmation of the validity of LNIT. *Methods:* A randomized, double-blind, placebo-controlled study of LNIT in patients allergic to *Parietaria* and *Dermathophagoides* was performed. Patients were evaluated, before and after treatment, with symptom and medication scores, specific nasal provocation tests, anterior rhinomanometry and mucociliary clearance time. *Results:* Compared to placebo the clinical efficacy of LNIT was confirmed by a reduction of clinical symptoms and drug intake. In the active group the reduction of allergen-specific nasal reactivity was significant. No local or systemic side effects were observed. *Conclusions:* The clinical efficacy of LNIT suggests that this therapy is effective in the prophylaxis of allergic rhinitis. Finally, there is no conflict between LNIT and drug treatment.

Introduction

Allergic rhinitis with a 20% incidence which is constantly increasing in relation to environmental (smog, cigarette smoke) and climatic factors is today considered a systemic disease with the nose as the 'shock organ' [1]. This trend has, consequently, resulted in an increase in social and economic expenditure on the disease arousing interest in prevention and, particularly, in specific immunosensitizing therapy administered subcutaneously or locally [2].

The aim of this therapy is to induce an increase in the title of specific IgG-blocking antibodies (particularly Ig4), a reduced lymphocyte proliferation response to the specific allergen, a growth of circulating CD8+ suppressor T cells, a gradual change in the differentiation of T lymphocytes with a switch from the T helper type 2 cells (which mainly produce interleukin 4) to the prevalent T helper type 1 cells (which produce interleukin 2 and interferon-γ). These changes in the lymphocyte cytokine profile induce a gradual reduction of IgE synthesis and inhibition of mast cell activation, thus impeding the release of the mediators of immune inflammation [3, 4].

The specific immunosensitizing therapy for the treatment of allergic diseases is the main etiological therapeutic tool, as demonstrated by many double-blind placebo-controlled clinical studies, recently reviewed by Abramson et al. [5] in a meta-analysis study. The efficacy of the treatment requires certain patient selection criteria, preparation and administration of hyposensitizing extracts. Its efficacy has been confirmed by double-blind clinical trials, reported in a World Health Organization Position Paper [6].

Relatively recently intranasal administration of the allergen has been adopted. In particular, specific local nasal immunosensitizing therapy (LNIT) that was first used by Herxheimer [1] in 1951 is based on direct immunotolerance induction in the shock organ with a reduced risk of side effects and costs. The standard treatment schedule consists of an induction phase with increasing dosages followed by a maintenance phase. Other treatment schedules consist of a constant dosage [7, 8].

It has been reported that LNIT reduces rhinitic symptoms and drug usage, as well as nasal reactivity towards the offending allergen. This study was designed to obtain further confirmation of the validity of LNIT in patients with allergic rhinitis monosensitive to perennial allergens (*Dermathophagoides*) or seasonal allergens (Graminaceae or *Parietaria*).

Material and Methods

Patients

Between February 1999 and July 2001, a total number of 96 patients (52 females, 44 males; mean age 31 years), suffering from nasal hyperreactivity symptoms, were enrolled from those attending our ENT Department. Inclusion and exclusion criteria were evaluated examining the description of clinical signs and symptoms, the morphological structure of nasal cavities, and causal factors.

The signs and symptoms considered were rhinorrhea, nasal obstruction and sneezing. The morphological structure of the nasal cavities was examined with anterior rhinoscopy. Skin prick tests, nasal provocation tests, nasal microbiological tests and mucociliary clearance time (MCT) were used to identify the causal factors. The skin prick tests were used to

Table 1. Distribution of patients undergoing LNIT

	Number	Active treatment	Placebo
LNIT mites	55	28 (11 M + 17 F)	27 (9 M + 18 F)
LNIT pollens	41	23 (13 M + 10 F)	18 (11 M + 7 F)

identify the inhaled allergens responsible for nasal allergies. The nasal provocation tests were performed in the case of pollens and mites using anterior rhinomanometry, as follows: baseline assessment to establish which nasal fossa had least resistance; insufflation of lactose powder into the nasal fossa that shows the lowest resistance and control with anterior active rhinomanometry; allergen challenge with doses of 2.5, 5, 10, 20, 40, 60, 80, 120, 160 and 240 allergen units (AU) at 10-min intervals, recording the rhinomanometric tracing at the end of each challenge. The test was considered positive for the allergen dose that caused an increase in resistance of 100% or more. The nasal microbiologial tests were done to identify concomitant infections. The MCT was measured by applying vegetable charcoal mixed with 3% saccharine to the mucosa at the medial face of the inferior turbinate. After patients were asked to breathe regularly and to report when they felt the sweet taste in their pharynx, an interval of 10–20 min was considered normal.

Patients were ineligible if they had skin prick tests or nasal provocation tests positive to more than one allergen; significant diseases or malformations of the nasal cavities such as nasal polyposis, septal deviation, choanal atresia; nasal swab positive for bacteria or mycetes, or immunotherapy in the preceding 5 years.

Criteria for inclusion in the study were no morphological alterations of nasal cavities; monosensitization to *Dermatophagoides*, grass or *Parietaria* pollens; nasal swab negative for bacteria or mycetes, or RAST positivity, at least class 3.

Of the 96 patients selected, 55 were positive for *Dermatophagoides* (57%) and 41 were positive for Graminaceae or *Parietaria* (43%). The patients selected were randomized into two groups: the active group that received specific LNIT and the placebo group that received a lactose powder formulation in order to be taste-masked. All patients gave written informed consent.

Each active product contained a single allergenic extract: from mites (*Dermatophagoides pteronyssinus* and *Dermatophagoides farinae*), from mixed Graminaceae (*Dactylis glomerata, Festuca elatior, Lolium italicum, Phleum pratense, Poa pratensis*) and from mixed *Parietaria* (*Parietaria judaica* and *Parietaria officinalis*), adsorbed on lactose, an inert excipient (table 1).

Dosage Schedule
The allergenic extracts were given every other day alternating between the two nostrils, according to the manufacture's schedule, at doses of 2.5, 5, 10, 20, 40, 60, 80, 120, 160 and 240 AU. Each dose was repeated 6 times until the highest dose had been given. Then the maintenance phase began during which every patient took the highest dose, 240 AU, weekly for 1 year alternating between the two nostrils.

Clinical and Instrumental Evaluation
Before treatment began and after 8 months of treatment patients graded the specific symptoms, nasal obstruction, sneezing and rhinorrhea, from 0 to 3 (0 = none; 1 = mild;

Table 2. LNIT for mites (symptoms before treatment)

Active treatment	Symptoms
Nasal obstruction	28
Rhinorrhea	23
Sneezing	18
Placebo	Symptoms
Nasal obstruction	25
Rhinorrhea	21
Sneezing	16

Table 3. LNIT for mites (symptoms after treatment)

	Active treatment			Placebo		
	nasal obstruction	rhinorrhea	sneezing	nasal obstruction	rhinorrhea	sneezing
Improved, %	82.1	65.2	55.5	12	19	18.8
Cured, %	7.2	17.4	27.7	0	0	0
No change, %	10.7	17.4	16.6	88	81	81.2
Responders, %	89.3	82.6	83.2	12	19	18.8
Responders, %		85			16.6	

2 = moderate; 3 = severe), according to their quality of life. During the follow-up, all patients had a monthly diary card where they entered the symptoms and the use of drugs.

The objective analysis was made with the nasal provocation test with the allergens, the nasal resistance measured by static and dynamic rhinomanometry at a preset pressure of 150 Pa in accordance with the recommendations of the International Standardization Committee [9], and MCT.

Results

During the treatment no patient had reported bronchospastic or systemic reactions. All patients completed their scheduled immunotherapy diaries and their signs and symptoms were classified into three categories: improvement, cured and no change.

Patients Allergic to Mites (tables 2, 3)
At the end of the trial, almost all LNIT patients (total = 28) reported a significant reduction of clinical signs. Active treatment revealed improvement of

Table 4. LNIT for pollens (symptoms before treatment)

	Symptoms
Active treatment	Symptoms
Nasal obstruction	22
Rhinorrhea	19
Sneezing	17
Placebo	Symptoms
Nasal obstruction	17
Rhinorrhea	15
Sneezing	14

Table 5. LNIT for pollens (symptoms after treatment)

	Active treatment			Placebo		
	nasal obstruction	rhinorrhea	sneezing	nasal obstruction	rhinorrhea	sneezing
Improved, %	68.2	63.1	52.9	23.5	20	14.3
Cured, %	9	21.1	29.4	0	0	0
No change, %	22.7	15.8	17.6	76.5	80	85.7
Responders, %	77.2	84.2	82.3	23.5	20	14.3
Responders, %		81.2			19.3	

nasal obstruction (total = 28) in 82.1% (n = 23), cure in 7.2% (n = 2), no change in 10.7% (n =3); improvement of rhinorrhea (total = 23) in 65.2% (n = 15), cure in 17.4% (n = 4), no change in 17.4% (n = 4), and improvement of sneezing (total = 18) in 55.5% (n = 10), cure in 27.7% (n = 5), no change in 16.6% (n = 3). The percentage of responders was 85%.

The placebo group showed improvement of nasal obstruction (total = 25) in 12% (n = 3), cure in 0% (n = 0), no change in 88% (n = 22); improvement of rhinorrhea (total = 21) in 19% (n = 4), cure in 0% (n = 0), no change in 81% (n = 17), and improvement of sneezing (n = 16) in 18.8% (n = 3), cure in 0% (n = 0), no change in 81.2% (n = 13). The percentage of responders was 16.6%.

Patients Allergic to Pollens (tables 4, 5)

At the end of the trial, almost all LNIT patients (total = 23) reported a significant reduction of clinical signs. Active treatment revealed improvement of nasal obstruction (total = 22) in 68.2% (n = 15), cure in 9% (n = 2),

Table 6. LNIT for mites (signs after treatment)

	Active treatment			Placebo		
	rhinomanometry	NPT	MCT	rhinomanometry	NPT	MCT
Improved, %	14.3	28.6	0	3.7	7.4	0
Cured, %	32.1	50	10.7	7.4	11.1	0
No change, %	53.6	21.4	89.3	88.9	81.5	100
Responders, %	46.4	78.6	10.7	11.1	18.5	0

NPT = Nasal provocation tests.

no change in 22.7% (n = 5); improvement of rhinorrhea (total = 19) in 63.1% (n = 12), cure in 21.1% (n = 4), no change in 15.8% (n = 3), and improvement of sneezing (total = 17) in 52.9% (n = 9), cure in 29.4% (n = 5), no change in 17.6% (n = 3). The percentage of responders was 81.2%.

The placebo group showed improvement of nasal obstruction (total = 17) in 23.5% (n = 4), cure in 0% (n = 0), no change in 76.5% (n = 13); improvement of rhinorrhea (total = 15) in 20% (n = 3), cure in 0% (n = 0), no change in 80% (n = 12), and improvement of sneezing (total = 14) in 14.3% (n = 2), cure in 0% (n = 0), no change in 85.7% (n = 12). The percentage of responders was 19.3%.

Instrumental Examination
Patients Allergic to Mites (table 6)
Rhinomanometry in the group of LNIT patients (n = 28) showed improvement in 14.3% (n = 4) and cure in 32.1% (n = 9) versus the placebo group (n = 27) that showed improvement in 3.7% (n = 1) and cure in 7.4% (n = 2). The nasal provocation test in the LNIT group showed a lowering of the threshold for reactivity in 78.6% (n = 22), improvement in 28.6% (n = 8) and cure in 50% (n = 12) compared with 7.4% (n = 2) and 11.1% (n = 3) of those given placebo. Mucociliary clearance time returned to normal in 10.7% (n = 3) of the LNIT group while none of those given placebo showed any improvement. The percentage of responders in the LNIT group was 45.2%, that in the placebo group 9.8%.

Patients Allergic to Pollens (table 7)
Rhinomanometry in the group of LNIT patients (n = 23) showed improvement in 21.7% (n = 5) and cure in 26.1% (n = 6) versus the placebo group (n = 18) that showed improvement in 0% (n = 0) and cure in 5.5% (n = 1).

Table 7. LNIT for pollens (signs after treatment)

	Active treatment			Placebo		
	rhinomanometry	NPT	MCT	rhinomanometry	NPT	MCT
Improved, %	21.7	21.7	0	0	11.1	0
Cured, %	26.1	30.5	8.7	5.5	5.6	0
No change, %	52.2	47.8	91.3	94.5	83.3	100
Responders, %	47.8	52.2	8.7	5.5	16.7	0

NPT = Nasal provocation tests.

The nasal provocation test in the LNIT group showed a lowering of the threshold for reactivity in 52.2% (n = 12), improvement in 21.7% (n = 5) and cure in 30.5% (n = 7) compared with 11.1% (n = 2) and 5.6% (n = 1) of those given placebo. Mucociliary clearance time returned to normal in 8.7% (n = 2) of the LNIT group while none of those given placebo showed any improvement. The percentage of responders in the LNIT group was 36.2%, that in the placebo group 7.4%.

Discussion

The indications for LNIT do not differ from those for the subcutaneous route of administration: LNIT should obviously be used in patients suffering from rhinitis, and its effectiveness seems to depend on the preseasonal administration. The possible local side effects do not, at present, represent a real problem.

During the last 15 years, a large number of controlled studies have provided evidence for the clinical effectiveness and safety of the LNIT [3, 10–25]. Position papers have evaluated the clinical use of LNIT based on a detailed and critical review of the literature. The clinical trials performed with LNIT are listed in table 8.

Our study confirms the clinical effectiveness of LNIT in reducing clinical symptoms and drug intake under natural allergen exposure. Specific LNIT appears to offer considerable advantages over other hyposensitization methods. As a matter of fact parenteral therapy is in many cases unsuccessful (incomplete and temporary) regarding recrudescence of symptoms, and, from an immunological point of view, produces a systemic immune response without interesting the local one of fundamental importance in upper airway reactivity.

Table 8. Clinical trials performed with LNIT

Authors and year of publication	Allergen	Type of extract	Duration	Patients	Significance
Johansson, 1979 [11]	grass	aqueous	14 weeks	12	<0.001
Nickelsen et al., 1981 [13]	ragweed	aqueous	3 months	38	<0.01
Welsh et al., 1981 [14]	ragweed	aqueous	20 weeks	18	<0.004
Schumacher and Pain, 1982 [12]	grass	powder	10 weeks	8	NS
Georgitis et al., 1986 [15]	grass	aqueous allergoid	10 weeks	15	<0.005
Andri et al., 1992 [16]	*Parietaria*	powder modified	18 weeks	8	NS
Passalacqua et al., 1995 [25]	*Parietaria*	powder	5 months	9	<0.01
D'Amato et al., 1995 [23]	*Parietaria*	powder	8 weeks	10	<0.05
Andri et al., 1996 [19]	grass	powder	16 weeks	13	<0.05
Motta et al., 2000 [3]	mites	powder	32 weeks	29	<0.0001

It can clearly be verified that any therapy, unable to influence the target organ's defense neurosis, is destined to have limited results [1].

Over the years there have been many failures with LNIT, due to the absence of standardization and the presence of local adverse reactions, particularly evident with the use of aqueous extracts. These inconvenients are synthesized in little stability (some molecules adhere to the inside surface of the container), autodigestion (presence of proteolytic enzymes in the extracts), and it is impossible to add propellants that enable their vaporization. It has become possible to overcome these problems after the realization of lyophilized allergenic preparations incorporated into an inert excipient in powder (lactose) and included in a rigid gelatine capsule [10, 26].

In addition, socioeconomic savings as a result of the self-administration of treatment (better patient compliance) should be taken into consideration.

Naturally the success of this therapeutic approach depends on the correct clinical investigation and on reliable diagnostic methods. For this reason in the evaluation of the efficacy of LNIT we include: nasal endoscopy ($0°$ diameter 4 mm; $30°$ diameter 2.7 mm), active anterior rhinomanometry, mucociliary transport time, specific nasal provocation test, and nasal microbiological test.

Equal importance must be attributed to the analysis of the clinical diaries of the patients regarding symptomatic scores, anti-H1 consumed, and general clinical judgement (improved, stationary, asymptomatic). Better results were obtained with allergies brought on by perennial allergens, then in seasonal ones due to pollens. This depends on the stage of the allergy at the beginning of the study. However, the active treatment was undoubtedly effective, especially as regards nasal obstruction. This was confirmed by the clinical diary and the rhinomanometric study.

Conclusions

The clinical efficacy of specific LNIT suggests that this therapy is effective as a prophylaxis in allergic rhinitis. This pathology must be studied primarily as a pathology specifically affecting the nose. The morphological and functional features of the nose must be borne in mind when choosing the treatment. It is equally important to identify the causes of allergic rhinitis. Our study confirms the efficacy and the advantages of LNIT with very few complications and better patient compliance.

The immunological modification induced by LNIT can be briefly summarized in the two points: (1) reduction of allergic symptoms and allergic phlogosis (decrease of local inflammatory cells) and (2) reduction of the provocative threshold with the specific nasal provocation test.

Correct clinical investigations and reliable diagnostic methods are of vital importance. Finally, there is no conflict between LNIT and drug treatment.

References

1   Passali D: Rinopatia vasomotoria specifica. Pisa, Pacini Editore, 1999.
2   D'Amato G, Bonini S, Bousquet J, Durham SR, Platts-Millis TAE: Pollenosis 2000: Global Approach. Napoli, JCC Editions, 2001.
3   Motta G, Passali D, De Vincentiis I, Ottavini A, Maurizi M, Sartoris A, Pallestrini E, Motta S, Salzano F: A multicenter trial of specific local nasal immunotherapy. Laryngoscope 2000;110: 132–139.
4   Passalacqua G, Albano M, Pronzato C, Riccio AM, Scordamaglia A, Falagiani P, Canonica GW: Long-term follow-up of nasal immunotherapy to Parietaria: Clinical and local immunological effects. Clin Exp Allergy 1997;27:904–908.
5   Abramson MJ, Puy RM, Weiner JM: Is allergen immunotherapy effective in asthma? Am Rev Respir Crit Care Med 1995;151:969–974.
6   Bousquet J, Lockey RF, Malling HJ: WHO Position Paper. Allergen immunotherapy: Therapeutic vaccines for allergic diseases. Allergy 1998(suppl 44):53.
7   Pocobelli D, Del Bono A, Venuti L, Venuti A, Falagiani P: Nasal immunotherapy at constant dosage: A double-blind, placebo-controlled study in grass-allergic rhinoconjunctivitis. J Investig Allergol Clin Immunol 2001;11/2:79–88.
8   Senna GE, Andri G, Dama AR, Falagiani P, Andri L: Local nasal immunotherapy: Efficacy and tolerability of two different administration schedules in grass pollen rhinitis. Allergol Immunopathol 2000;28:238–242.
9   Clement PAR: Committee report on standardization of rhinomanometry. Rhinology 1984;22: 151–155.

10 Marcucci F, Sensi LG, Caffarelli C, Cavagni G, Bernardini R, Tiri A, Riva G, Novembre E: Low-dose local nasal immunotherapy in children with perennial allergic rhinitis due to Dermatophagoides. Allergy 2002;57/1:23–28.

11 Johansson SGO, Deuschl H, Zetterström O: Use of glutaraldehyde-modified timothy grass pollen extract in nasal hyposensitization treatment of hay fever. Int Arch Allergy Appl Immunol 1979; 60:447–460.

12 Schumacher MJ, Pain MC: Intranasal immunotherapy and polymerized grass pollen allergens. Allergy 1982;37:241–248.

13 Nickelsen JA, Goldstein S, Mueller U: Local intranasal immunotherapy for ragweed allergic rhinitis. I. Clinical response. J Allergy Clin Immunol 1981;68:33–40.

14 Welsh PW, Zimmermann EM, Yunginger JW, Kern EB, Gleich GJ: Preseasonal intranasal immunotherapy with nebulized shot ragweed extract. J Allergy Clin Immunol 1981;67:237–242.

15 Georgitis JW, Nickelsen JA, Wypych J, Barde SH, Clayton WF, Reisman RE: Local intranasal immunotherapy with high dose polymerized ragweed extract. Int Arch Allergy Appl Immunol 1986;81:170–173.

16 Andri L, Senna GE, Betteli C, Givanni S, Andri G, Falagiani P, Lugo G: Local nasal immunotherapy in allergic rhinitis to Parietaria. A double-blind controlled study. Allergy 1992;47:318–323.

17 Andri L, Senna GE, Betteli C, Givanni S, Andri G, Falagiani P: Local nasal immunotherapy for Dermatophagoides-induced rhinitis: Efficacy of a powder extract. J Allergy Clin Immunol 1993; 91:987–996.

18 Andri L, Senna GE, Andri G: Local nasal immunotherapy for birch allergic rhinitis with extract in powder form. Clin Exp Allergy 1995;25:1092–1099.

19 Andri L, Senna GE, Betteli G: Local nasal immunotherapy with extract in powder form is effective and safe in grass pollen rhinitis: A double-blind study. J Allergy Clin Immunol 1996;97: 34–41.

20 Cirla A, Sforza N, Roffi G: Preseasonal intranasal immunotherapy in birch-alder allergic rhinitis. A double-blind study. Allergy 1996;51:299–306.

21 Bardare M, Zani G, Novembre E, Vierucci A: Local nasal immunotherapy with a powdered extract for grass pollen-induced rhinitis in pediatric age. J Investig Allergol Clin Immunol 1996;6:359–363.

22 Ariano R, Panzani RC, Chiapella M, Augeri G, Falagiani P: Local immunotherapy of seasonal allergic rhinitis in children due to *Parietaria officinalis* pollen. A preliminary report. Pediatr Asthma Allergy Immunol 1993;7/4:227–237.

23 D'Amato G, Lobefalo G, Liccardi G, Cazzola M: A double-blind, placebo-controlled trial of local nasal immunotherapy in allergic rhinitis to Parietaria pollen. Clin Exp Allergy 1995;25:141–148.

24 Ariano R, Panzani RC, Chiapella M, Augeri G, Falagiani P: Local intranasal immunotherapy with allergen in powder in atopic patients sensitive to *Parietaria officinalis* pollen. J Investig Allergol Clin Immunol 1995;5:126–132.

25 Passalacqua G, Albano M, Ruffoni S: Nasal immunotherapy to Parietaria: Evidence of reduction of local allergic inflammation. Am J Respir Crit Care Med 1995;152:461–466.

26 Passalacqua G, Bagnasco M, Mariani G, Falagiani P, Canonica GW: Local immunotherapy: Pharmacokinetics and efficacy. EAACI/PTA Symposium Reviews. Allergy 1998;53:477–484.

Dir. Prof. Gaetano Motta
Clinica Otorinolaringoiatrica, Seconda Università di Napoli,
Ospedale Gesù e Maria, Via Cotugno 3, I–80135 Napoli (Italy)
Tel. +39 81 5666261, Fax +39 81 5666263, E-Mail gae.motta@libero.it

Markert UR, Elsner P (eds): Local Immunotherapy in Allergy.
Chem Immunol Allergy. Basel, Karger, 2003, vol 82, pp 99–108

·······················

Nonspecific Plasma Proteins during Sublingual Immunotherapy

M. Reich[a,b], *G. Zwacka*[c], *U.R. Markert*[a,b]

[a]Department of Dermatology and Allergology and [b]Department of Obstetrics,
Friedrich Schiller University, Jena, and [c]Children's Hospital, Robert Koch Hospital,
Apolda, Germany

Key Words

Sublingual immunotherapy · Allergy · Interleukin-2 receptor · Soluble intercellular
adhesion molecule-1 · Immunoglobulin G4 · sE-selectin · Interleukin · Immunoglobulin E

Abstract

Usually, specific allergy-related plasma proteins such as immunoglobulin E (IgE) and
immunoglobulin G (IgG) are used for estimating the grade of sensitization and follow-up
of immunotherapy. In recent years, several nonspecific inflammatory markers, such as
sICAM-1 and sIL-2R, have been shown as being suitable for therapy control in allergy. In
our investigation of patients under sublingual immunotherapy (SLIT), plasma from 42
healthy controls and 133 children with single inhalation allergies to grass pollen, birch
pollen or house dust mites was obtained during the symptom-free period. Patients showed
symptoms including allergic rhinitis, dermatitis and allergic asthma with one single RAST
class 3 or higher. Plasma concentrations of soluble intercellular adhesion molecule-1
(sICAM-1), soluble interleukin-2 receptor (sIL-2R), sE-selectin, interleukin-12 (IL-12) and
specific IgG4 were analyzed with the ELISA technique. After 1 year of SLIT, concentrations of sICAM-1, sIL-2R and sE-selectin declined significantly when results from all
patients were taken as one group. Regarding the single allergen groups, the sICAM-1 and
sIL-2R decrease was significant in the grass and mite group, but not in the birch group,
while the sE-selectin decline was only significant in the birch group after 1 year of SLIT,
but not in the grass and the mite group. No difference was observed in IL-12 and IgG4
expression. In two groups of controls with a mean age of 9.5 versus 17.5 years, the analyzed
parameters were not age-dependent. The increased proteins may be useful as additional
markers for the evaluation of immunological effects and follow-up investigations of allergy
therapies.

Introduction

Different methods are routinely used for diagnosis and monitoring of atopic diseases. On the one hand, there are the classical skin tests like the skin prick test and on the other, the more modern methods like the measurement of specific immunoglobulin E (IgE) or immunoglobulin G4 (IgG4) in the patients' plasma. Standardized questionnaires are available for the documentation of symptoms, medications and evaluation of the quality of life. Additionally to these established procedures, markers are investigated, which could contribute to analyzing the efficacy and mechanisms of therapies in allergies or to understanding the mechanisms of atopic disorders. For reasons of practicability, these markers should be easily analyzable in daily routine practice.

For the present open observation on sublingual immunotherapy (SLIT), nonspecific inflammatory markers were chosen, which are supposed to be involved in the allergic cascade and which can be measured by common ELISA techniques: soluble intercellular adhesion molecule-1 (sICAM-1), sE-selectin, soluble interleukin-2 receptor (sIL-2R), interleukin-12 (IL-12) and specific IgG4. Earlier investigations in this field were mostly performed on a smaller number of patients and the results are sometimes contradicting.

ICAM-1 (CD54) is physiologically expressed on the surface of antigen-presenting cells (APC) and activated vessels. It enables APC to contact T cells and prolongs their time of stay. The soluble form sICAM-1 probably has its origin in the membrane-bound cell surface homologue and is not separately secreted [1]. IL-2R is expressed on the surface of helper and cytotoxic T cells, B cells, neutrophils, monocytes and other cells. The IL-2R construct is unique among the growth factor receptors because it consists of an α-, β- and γ-chain (CD25, CD122, CD132) with different functions. Nonactivated T cells express only the β- and γ-chain. Antigen recognition and costimulation initiate the expression of the α-chain, which leads to an enormous increase in receptor affinity [for review, see 2]. The 10-kD smaller soluble form sIL-2R is shed from the cell surface and can be detected in the plasma [3]. E-selectin (CD62E) is expressed on vascular endothelium. It takes part in the homing process of T lymphocytes, but for passing through the vessel wall, further adhesion molecules like the integrins are necessary [4]. IL-12 is produced mainly by APC and is a strong inducer of a Th1 answer after antigen challenge. Although IgG4 amounts to only 4% of the total IgG, it can be elevated in allergic individuals undergoing immunotherapy. The exact mode of action and its natural function is still unknown. Concerning immunotherapy, it may work as a blocking antibody [5].

The aim of the present investigation was to analyze immunological effects of SLIT by monitoring the mentioned plasma proteins.

Methods

Patients/Blood Samples

The investigated blood samples were obtained from allergic outpatients of the Children's Hospital, Apolda, Germany. All analyses were performed at the Friedrich Schiller University, Jena. From a total of 133 different patients 309 samples were analyzed: 62 derived from birch, 154 from grass and 93 from mite-sensitive children. The mean age was 12 years (SD 5.4 years).

The including criteria were one single RAST class between 3 and 6 and a certain diagnosis. The blood samples were taken outside the allergen season or in the low symptom period for mites. At that time no acute allergic exacerbation or no other inflammatory disease was apparent. Patients sensitive to more than one allergen or with an airway remodeling in asthma were excluded. A signed consent from the parents was required before starting the analyses.

ELISA

Plasma was separated from heparinized blood samples, aliquoted and stored at $-80°C$. All samples were then analyzed simultaneously with identical batches of antibodies and other reagents. ELISAs for the detection of sICAM-1, sE-selectin and IL-12 were performed with ELI-Pairs (Diaclone, France; distributed by Hölzel, Germany). 96-well Maxisorp plates (Nunc) were coated overnight with capture antibodies at 4°C. After 1 h sample incubation, detection was performed with biotinylated anti-ICAM-1, anti-sE-selectin or anti IL-12 detection antibodies followed by streptavidin-horse raddish peroxidase and a TMB color reaction. Light absorption was detected with a Spectra ELISA reader at 450 nm.

Complete commercial ELISA kits containing coated plates were used for the detection of sIL-2R (kind gift from DPC Biermann) and IgG4 (Hycor Biomedical). Detection and color reaction were analogous to that mentioned earlier. All tests were performed in duplicate wells.

Statistics

All data were analyzed as paired samples using the Wilcoxon test. For all calculations, SPSS software was used.

Results

Estimation of Age Dependency

To avoid age-dependent results all controls were divided into two groups: the older 50% and the younger 50%. Mean age of the younger controls was 9.5 years versus 17.5 years in the older controls. There was no difference between these groups, indicating no age dependency of the analyzed parameters in adolescence (data not shown).

sICAM-1

Median plasma levels of sICAM-1 were significantly higher before starting SLIT (805.0 ng/ml) compared with levels during therapy (1 year 723.3 ng/ml,

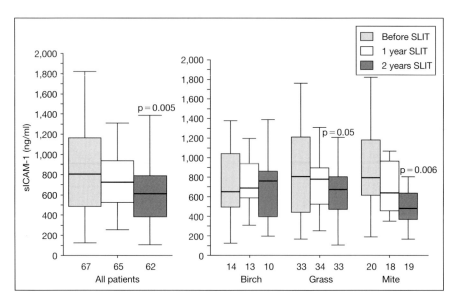

Fig. 1. Box plots of sICAM-1 plasma levels of patients before and during SLIT. When changes were significant compared with values before therapy, p is given. Left plots show values for all patients. Right plots show groups formed according to the respective allergen.

2 years 612.0 ng/ml). Regarding the single allergy groups the decrease of the levels was significant in patients with grass pollen allergy (805.3 to 671.7 ng/ml) and house dust mite allergy (794.2 to 479.7 ng/ml) after 2 years of SLIT (see fig. 1).

sIL-2R

Median levels of sIL-2R were significantly higher before SLIT (596.7 U/ml; 1 year's SLIT: 371.4 U/ml; 2 years' SLIT: 345.6 U/ml). Also, in all single allergy groups, sIL-2R plasma levels were reduced. This reduction was significant only in patients sensitive to grass pollen (before: 592.3 U/ml; 1 year: 366.9 U/ml; 2 years: 348.3 U/ml) and mites (before: 564.7 U/ml; 1 year: 395.0 U/ml; 2 years: 327.5 U/ml) (see fig. 2).

sE-Selectin

The median plasma concentration of sE-selectin of all patients was 158.5 ng/ml before starting SLIT. After the 1st year of therapy, the median sE-selectin level was 126.2 ng/ml and after another year, 137.6 ng/ml, which are both a significant decline compared with the starting point. Concerning the

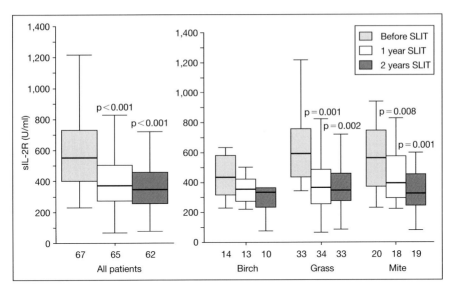

Fig. 2. Box plots of sIL-2R plasma levels of patients before and during SLIT. When changes were significant compared with values before therapy, p is given. Left plots show values for all patients. Right plots show groups formed according to the respective allergen.

single allergy groups, the decrease was obvious but not significant except in the birch pollen group in the 1st year of therapy (see fig. 3).

IL-12

IL-12 levels declined during the 1st year under SLIT. After 2 years, the plasma level is slightly, but not significantly, elevated compared to the starting point (fig. 4).

Specific IgG4

The results of the semiquantitative ELISA show a very slightly but not significantly higher rate of increase than of decrease (see fig. 5). In approximately 80% of patients no change was detectable.

Discussion

Earlier results from our group with a large number of 133 allergic patients demonstrate elevated levels in various inflammatory plasma proteins [6]. Some of those patients now show a clear decrease during SLIT, which is significant for sICAM-1, sIL-2R and sE-selectin. Regarding the single groups, classified

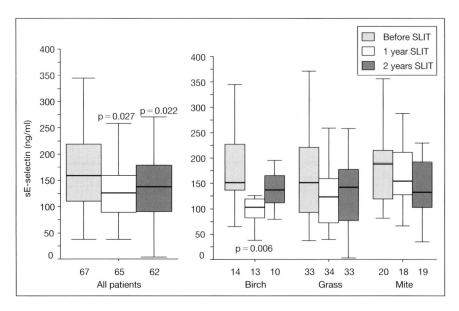

Fig. 3. Box plots of sE-selectin plasma levels of patients before and during SLIT. When changes were significant compared with values before therapy, p is given. Left plots show values for all patients. Right plots show groups formed according to the respective allergen.

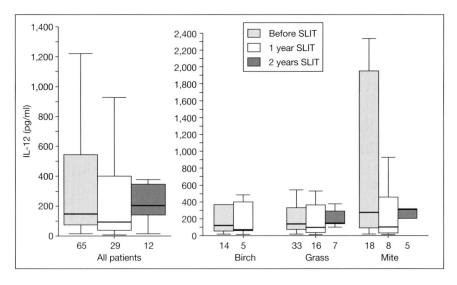

Fig. 4. Box plots of IL-12 plasma levels of patients before and during SLIT. When changes were significant compared with values before therapy, p is given. Left plots show values for all patients. Right plots show groups formed according to the respective allergen.

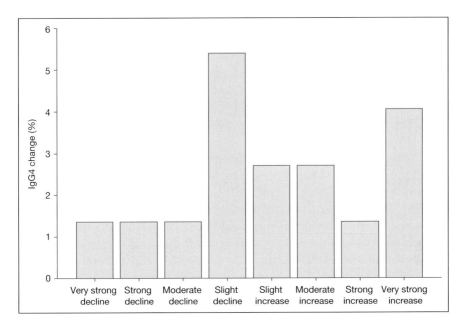

Fig. 5. Specific IgG4 was analyzed by using a commercially available semiquantitative ELISA, which was able to classify values into four groups. Changes towards lower or higher categories were counted. The figures demonstrate the changes of plasma levels of the respective specific IgG4 during SLIT as in percent of all patients. In approximately 80% of patients no change was observed.

according to the causative allergens (grass, birch or mites), the plasma levels decreased significantly in some, but not all groups, which might be due to the lower number of patients.

Several studies are published using the above mentioned plasma proteins as markers for allergy follow-up during subcutaneous immunotherapy partly with contradicting results. sICAM-1 has been shown to be elevated in allergic rhinitis, conjunctivitis and asthma [7–10]. During SIT, a significant decrease of sICAM-1 was described in grass pollen allergy [11] and in seasonal and perennial allergic rhinitis [12–14]. Until now, observations on sE-selectin plasma concentrations have not yet been published. Thus far, only differences between untreated allergic patients and healthy controls were investigated. sE-selectin plasma levels were elevated in most of these observations in allergic individuals [15–21], but decreased levels were also reported in one study [22]. Furthermore, the results of published analyses of sIL-2R plasma levels are inhomogeneous. Especially in patients with allergic asthma or atopic dermatitis, sIL-2R plasma levels were increased [23–25]. It has been described elsewhere that such an elevation occurred only during the season, which was reduced in patients responding well to SIT [13]. In perennial allergic rhinitis caused by *Dermatophagoides farinae*, a decreased sIL-2R and an increased IgG4 level after a therapy period of 3 years have been shown, which correlated with the clinical improvement [26]. 10 years after therapy, sICAM-1 was still significantly reduced [26]. Another study investigated patients allergic to house dust mites and found significantly elevated sIL-2R as well as IL-2 concentrations compared with healthy controls. The values normalized after 3 years of SIT [23].

Although former investigations demonstrated an influence of IL-12 on the establishment of a Th1 pattern during immunotherapies, in our hands no changes became obvious [27, 28].

In contrast to the above-mentioned proteins, IgG4 is a molecule which reacts specifically with the allergen and therefore undoubtedly interacts with allergic disorders, although its exact role is still discussed controversely. Some studies describe increased specific IgG4 during SLIT and interpret this in analogy to experience with the subcutaneous form as therapeutic success [29–33]. Other authors demonstrate stable IgG4 levels [34–36]. A study showing that a high IgG4 antibody level is associated with a failure of the immunotherapy with inhalant allergens is difficult to interpret with the current concepts [37]. Summarizing the data on IgG4, its role as a marker of success or failure of immunotherapies cannot yet be conclusively answered. Further investigations and more details concerning its function in allergies are necessary.

In general, the present results indicate an nonspecific inflammatory reaction in allergy. The expression of the proteins analyzed, at least in their soluble form, may change more as an epiphenomenon of allergy than contribute causatively to the sensitization or effector process. Although their implication in plasma remains unclear, their concentrations may serve as markers for the evaluation of the accompanying inflammation of an allergic disorder.

It is not clear yet whether any of the investigated parameters can be used for new diagnostic aspects of individual patients, but it can, at least, be used for observation and follow-up investigations of groups of patients. The analysis of plasma level progression, especially of sICAM-1, sIL-2R and sE-selectin, provides an additional aspect in the evaluation of allergy therapies and their functional mechanisms.

References

1   Rothlein R, Mainolfi EA, Czajkowsi M, Marlin SD: A form of circulating ICAM-1 in human serum. J Immunol 1991;147:3488–3493.
2   Minami Y, Kono T, Miyazaki T, Taniguchi T: The IL-2 receptor complex: Its structure, function, and target genes. Annu Rev Immunol 1993;11:245–268.

3 Honda M, Kitamura K, Takeshita T, Sugamura K, Tokunaga T: Identification of a soluble IL-2 receptor beta-chain from human lymphoid cell line cells. J Immunol 1990;145:4131–4135.

4 Binns RM, Licence ST, Harrison AA, Keelan ET, Robinson MK, Haskard DO: In vivo E-selectin upregulation correlates early with infiltration of PMN, later with PBL entry: MAbs block both. Am J Physiol 1996;270:183–193.

5 Oehling A, Sanz ML, Garcia BE: Immunological parameters in the immunotherapy follow-up. Int Arch Allergy Immunol 1992;99:474–477.

6 Reich M, Niess JH, Bär C, Zwacka G, Markert UR: Elevated non-specific plasma proteins in allergic patients. J Investig Allergol Clin Exp, in press.

7 El Sawy IH, Badr El Din OM, El Azzouni OE, Motawae HA: Soluble intercellular adhesion molecule-1 in sera of children with bronchial asthma exacerbation. Int Arch Allergy Immunol 1999;119:126–132.

8 Cengizlier R, Demirpolat E, Tulek N, Cakmak F: Circulating ICAM-1 levels in bronchial asthma and the effect of inhaled corticosteroids. Ann Allergy Asthma Immunol 2000;84:539–541.

9 Hashimoto S, Imai K, Kobayashi T, Amemiya E, Takahashi Y, Tomita Y, Iwata T, Suguro H, Yamaguchi M, Yachi A: Elevated levels of soluble ICAM-1 in sera from patients with bronchial asthma. Allergy 1993;48:370–372.

10 Wuthrich B, Joller-Jemelka H, Kagi MK: Levels of soluble ICAM-1 in atopic dermatitis. A new marker for monitoring the clinical activity? Allergy 1995;50:88–89.

11 Passalacqua G, Senna G, Dama A, Riccio A, Crivellaro M, Canonica GW: The relationship between clinical efficacy of specific immunotherapy and serum intercellular adhesion molecule-1 levels. J Investig Allergol Clin Immunol 1998;8:123–124.

12 Ohashi Y, Nakai Y, Tanaka A, Kakinoki Y, Ohno Y, Masamoto T, Sakamoto H, Kato A, Washio Y, Yamada K, Hayashi M: Clinical role of soluble adhesion molecules during immunotherapy for perennial allergic rhinitis. Arch Otolaryngol Head Neck Surg 1998;124:41–45.

13 Ohashi Y, Nakai Y, Tanaka A, Kakinoki Y, Ohno Y, Masamoto T, Sakamoto H, Kato A, Washio Y, Hayashi M: Serum levels of specific IgE, soluble interleukin-2 receptor, and soluble intercellular adhesion molecule-1 in seasonal allergic rhinitis. Ann Allergy Asthma Immunol 1997;79: 213–220.

14 Ohashi Y, Nakai Y, Tanaka A, Kakinoki Y, Ohno Y, Masamoto T, Sakamoto H, Kato A, Washio Y, Hayashi M: Soluble intercellular adhesion molecule-1 level in sera is elevated in perennial allergic rhinitis. Laryngoscope 1997;107:932–935.

15 Yamashita N, Kaneko S, Kouro O, Furue M, Yamamoto S, Sakane T: Soluble E-selectin as a marker of disease activity in atopic dermatitis. J Allergy Clin Immunol 1997;99:410–416.

16 Wolkerstorfer A, Laan MP, Savelkoul HF, Neijens HJ, Mulder PG, Oudesluys-Murphy AM, Sukhai RN, Oranje AP: Soluble E-selectin, other markers of inflammation and disease severity in children with atopic dermatitis. Br J Dermatol 1998;138:431–435.

17 Koide M, Furukawa F, Tokura Y, Shirahama S, Takigawa M: Evaluation of soluble cell adhesion molecules in atopic dermatitis. J Dermatol 1997;24:88–93.

18 Hirai S, Kageshita T, Kimura T, Tsujisaki M, Okajima K, Imai K, Ono T: Soluble intercellular adhesion molecule-1 and soluble E-selectin levels in patients with atopic dermatitis. Br J Dermatol 1996;134:657–661.

19 Czech W, Schopf E, Kapp A: Soluble E-selectin in sera of patients with atopic dermatitis and psoriasis – Correlation with disease activity. Br J Dermatol 1996;134:17–21.

20 Morita H, Kitano Y, Kawasaki N: Elevation of serum-soluble E-selectin in atopic dermatitis. J Dermatol Sci 1995;10:145–150.

21 Kowalzick L, Kleinheinz A, Neuber K, Weichenthal M, Kohler I, Ring J: Elevated serum levels of soluble adhesion molecules ICAM-1 and ELAM-1 in patients with severe atopic eczema and influence of UVA1 treatment. Dermatology 1995;190:14–18.

22 Laan MP, Koning H, Baert MR, Oranje AP, Buurman WA, Savelkoul HF, Neijens HJ: Levels of soluble intercellular adhesion molecule-1, soluble E-selectin, tumor necrosis factor-alpha, and soluble tumor necrosis factor receptor p55 and p75 in atopic children. Allergy 1998;53: 51–58.

23 Tsai LC, Tang RB, Hung MW, Chen HM, Tsai SJ: Expression of serum IL-2, IL-2R, and CD8 levels during hyposensitization in house-dust-sensitive asthmatics. J Asthma 1990;27:307–313.

24 Shi HZ, Sun JJ, Pan HL, Lu JQ, Zhang JL, Jiang JD: Alterations of T-lymphocyte subsets, soluble IL-2 receptor, and IgE in peripheral blood of children with acute asthma attacks. J Allergy Clin Immunol 1999;103:388–394.

25 Ohashi Y, Nakai Y, Sakamoto H, Ohno Y, Sugiura Y, Okamoto H, Tanaka A, Kakinoki Y, Kishimoto K, Hayashi M: Serum levels of soluble interleukin-2 receptor in patients with perennial allergic rhinitis before and after immunotherapy. Ann Allergy Asthma Immunol 1996;77:203–208.

26 Ohashi Y, Nakai Y, Tanaka A, Kakinoki Y, Washio Y, Kato A, Masamoto T, Sakamoto H, Yamada K: Ten-year follow-up study of allergen-specific immunoglobulin E and immunoglobulin G4, soluble interleukin-2 receptor, interleukin-4, soluble intercellular adhesion molecule-1 and soluble vascular cell adhesion molecule-1 in serum of patients on immunotherapy for perennial allergic rhinitis. Scand J Immunol 1998;47:167–178.

27 Lee YL, Fu CL, Ye YL, Chiang BL: Administration of interleukin 12 prevents mite Der p 1 allergen-IgE antibody production and airway eosinophil infiltration in an animal model of airway inflammation. Scand J Immunol 1999;49:229–236.

28 Gavett SH, O'Hearn DJ, Li X, Huang SK, Finkelman FD, Wills-Karp M: Interleukin 12 inhibits antigen-induced airway hyperresponsiveness, inflammation, and Th2 cytokine expression in mice. J Exp Med 1995;182:1527–1536.

29 Fanta C, Bohle B, Hirt W, Siemann U, Horak F, Kraft D, Ebner H, Ebner C: Systemic immunological changes induced by administration of grass pollen allergens via the oral mucosa during sublingual immunotherapy. Int Arch Allergy Immunol 1999;120:218–224.

30 Bousquet J, Scheinmann P, Guinnepain MT, Perrin Fayolle M, Sauvaget J, Tonnel AB, Pauli G, Caillaud D, Dubost R, Leynadier F, Vervloet D, Herman D, Galvain S, Andre C: Sublingual-swallow immunotherapy (SLIT) in patients with asthma due to house-dust mites: A double-blind, placebo-controlled study. Allergy 1999;54:249–260.

31 La Rosa M, Ranno C, Andre C, Carat F, Tosca MA, Canonica GW: Double-blind placebo-controlled evaluation of sublingual-swallow immunotherapy with standardized *Parietaria judaica* extract in children with allergic rhinoconjunctivitis. J Allergy Clin Immunol 1999;104:425–432.

32 Clavel R, Bousquet J, Andre C: Clinical efficacy of sublingual-swallow immunotherapy: A double-blind, placebo-controlled trial of a standardized five-grass-pollen extract in rhinitis. Allergy 1998;53:493–498.

33 Mungan D, Misirligil Z, Gurbuz L: Comparison of the efficacy of subcutaneous and sublingual immunotherapy in mite-sensitive patients with rhinitis and asthma – A placebo controlled study. Ann Allergy Asthma Immunol 1999;82:485–490.

34 Ambrosio F, Ricciardi L, Isola S, Savi E, Parmiani S, Puccinelli P, Musarra A: Rush sublingual immunotherapy in Parietaria allergic patients. Allergol Immunopathol (Madr) 1996;24:146–151.

35 Vourdas D, Syrigou E, Potamianou P, Carat F, Batard T, Andre C, Papageorgiou PS: Double-blind, placebo-controlled evaluation of sublingual immunotherapy with standardized olive pollen extract in pediatric patients with allergic rhinoconjunctivitis and mild asthma due to olive pollen sensitization. Allergy 1998;53:662–672.

36 Guez S, Vatrinet C, Fadel R, Andre C: House-dust-mite sublingual-swallow immunotherapy (SLIT) in perennial rhinitis: A double-blind, placebo-controlled study. Allergy 2000;55:369–375.

37 Djurup R, Malling HJ: High IgG4 antibody level is associated with failure of immunotherapy with inhalant allergens. Clin Allergy 1987;17:459–468.

Dr. Udo R. Markert, Abteilung für Geburtshilfe,
Friedrich-Schiller-Universität, D–07740 Jena (Germany)
Tel. +49 3641 933763, Fax +49 3641 933764, E-Mail udo.markert@med.uni-jena.de

Markert UR, Elsner P (eds): Local Immunotherapy in Allergy.
Chem Immunol Allergy. Basel, Karger, 2003, vol 82, pp 109–118

....

Safety of Allergen-Specific Sublingual Immunotherapy and Nasal Immunotherapy

Giovanni Passalacqua, Federica Fumagalli, Laura Guerra,
Giorgio Walter Canonica

Allergy and Respiratory Diseases, Department of Internal Medicine,
Genoa University, Genoa, Italy

Key Words

Sublingual immunotherapy · Local nasal immunotherapy · Safety · Side effects

Abstract

Allergen-specific immunotherapy is a well-established treatment for respiratory allergy. It is usually administered subcutaneously, and with this route several severe adverse events and fatalities have been described. Therefore, in the last 15 years, novel routes of administration (local routes) were developed. Sublingual and local nasal immunotherapy are now considered as viable alternatives to the injection route, mainly due to their optimal safety. The use of nasal immunotherapy is at present declining. On the other hand, sublingual immunotherapy was investigated in twenty-two randomized controlled trials and two post-marketing surveys: its safety profile turned out to be satisfactory in both adults and children, gastrointestinal complaints being the most frequently reported side effects. These side effects were always mild and could be treated with proper dose adjusting. At variance with injection immunotherapy, no severe systemic adverse event has ever been described. Its safety is also supported by pharmacokinetics and immunological data. Experimental data on the safety of sublingual and nasal immunotherapy will be reviewed.

The Question of Safety: Historical Background of Sublingual and Nasal Immunotherapy

Allergen-specific immunotherapy (IT) is the practice of administering increasing amounts of allergens to allergic subjects in order to achieve a hyposensitization and to reduce the symptoms during the natural exposure to the allergen itself. Since the first empirical attempts made by Leonard Noon [1], the allergenic extracts were administered subcutaneously (subcutaneous immunotherapy, SCIT). Indeed the encouraging positive results immediately led to a widespread use of the treatment, which was frequently unsuitable or incorrect. The idea of administering the allergenic extracts by routes other than the subcutaneous one is not recent: the first attempts with the oral route were made at the beginning of the last century [2, 3]. During the 1950s several trials with local bronchial IP were published [4]; in the 1970s some studies focused on the local nasal immunotherapy (LNIT) [5] and in the 1980s the sublingual route was proposed. All these approaches remained anecdotal and of speculative interest only, since the use of the subcutaneous route was well established and supported.

In the middle of the 1980s, the British Committee for the Safety of Medicines [6] reported twenty-six deaths clearly caused by injection IT, thus raising serious concerns about the safety and the risk/benefit ratio of IT and also in view of the fact that at the time increasingly more effective drugs were available. Subsequently, a detailed analysis of the literature demonstrated that most of the life-threatening or fatal events were, in principle, avoidable [7–9], but the interest in the noninjection routes of IT rapidly increased. In fact, the primary aim of these routes is minimizing the risk of adverse events and improving the acceptance by the patients [10]. In 1998 a panel of experts of the World Health Organization, based on an extensive review of the literature, concluded that only sublingual (SLIT) and local nasal (LNIT) IT are acceptable in the clinical practice [11]. These conclusions were confirmed in another position paper prepared by the European Academy of Allergology and Clinical Immunology (EAACI) [12]. In these documents, the indications were limited to adult patients, since the safety in children was considered not to have been sufficiently investigated. Meanwhile, postmarketing surveillance studies and new clinical trials appeared and, in 2001, the ARIA position paper also accepted the use of SLIT in pediatric patients [13]. The effectiveness and safety of the nasal route (LNIT) is supported by 14 double-blind placebo-controlled studies [12, 13]. Nevertheless, LNIT is only effective regarding rhinitis symptoms, it requires a particular administration technique, and it is difficult to give it to children; therefore, its use is progressively decreasing. LNIT is still used in a minority of patients as preseasonal treatment for pollenosis. At present, SLIT (sublingual-swallow) is the most extensively used and investigated route.

Experimental Evidence: Safety of SLIT in the Controlled Trials

The first data evaluating the safety of SLIT obviously come from the controlled clinical trials, which are, in turn, designed to assess the efficacy of

Table 1. Sublingual Immunotherapy Double Blind Placebo Controlled studies

Authors, year	Age range	Allergen	Duration	Cumulative dose	Patients[1]	Disease
Tari et al., 1990 [14]	5–12	mites	18 months	365 STU	30/28	R/A
Sabbah et al., 1994 [15]	13–51	grasses	17 weeks	4,500 IR	19/29	R
Feliziani et al., 1995 [17]	14–48	grasses	3.5 months	25 BU	18/16	R
Troise et al., 1995 [16]	17–60	*Parietaria*	10 months	105 BU	15/16	R
Hirsch et al., 1997 [18]	6–16	mites	1 year	570 µg Der p 1	15/15	R/A
Passalacqua et al., 1998 [23]	15–46	mites	2 years	10,000 AU	10/9	R
Vourdas et al., 1998 [21]	7–17	olive	2 years	4 mg Ole e 1	33/31	R/A
Clavel et al., 1998 [19]	8–55	grasses	6 months	28 µg Phl p 5	62/28	R/A
Horak et al., 1998 [20]	16–48	birch	4 months	250 STU	18/16	R
Hordijk et al., 1998 [22]	18–45	grasses	6 months	100,000 BU	30/27	R/A
Bousquet et al., 1999 [25]	15–37	mites	2 years	25 mg Der p 1	15/15	A
Passalacqua et al., 1999 [24]	15–42	*Parietaria*	8 months	16 µg Par j 1	15/15	R/A
Pradalier et al., 1999 [27]	6–25	grasses	4 months	5,000 STU	59/61	R/A
La Rosa et al., 1999 [28]	6–14	*Parietaria*	6 months	4,000 STU	20/21	R/A
Purello et al., 1999 [26]	14–50	*Parietaria*	8 months	12 µg Par j 1	14/16	R/A
Pajno et al., 2000 [30]	8–15	mites	2 years	2.4 mg Der p 1	12/12	A
Guez et al., 2000 [29]	6–51	mites	2 years	2.2 mg Der p 1	24/18	R
Caffarelli et al., 2000 [31]	4–14	grasses	3 months	32,000 AU	24/20	R/A
Ariano et al., 2001 [32]	19–50	cypress	8 months	250,000 RU	10/10	R/A
Bahceciler et al., 2001 [33]	7–15	mites	6 months	2,000 IR	8/7	R/A
Voltolini et al., 2001 [34]	15–52	trees	24 months	4,000 IR	24/13	R
Lima et al., 2002 [35]	16–48	grasses	18 months	16 mg Phl p 5	24/22	R

R = Rhinitis; A = asthma; STU = standard units; IR = index of reactivity; BU = biological units; AU = allergenic units; RU = rast units.
[1] Active/placebo.

the treatment as a primary outcome. The available literature on SLIT has been reviewed according to the restrictive criteria established by WHO and EAACI [11, 12]: only double-blind placebo-controlled trials published in peer-reviewed journals and with adequate methods and statistical analysis are considered. At present, there are twenty-two randomized, double-blind placebo-controlled clinical trials of SLIT [14–35] as summarized in table 1. Seven of these studies were performed in pediatric patients [18, 21, 28–31, 33].

Looking at the studies, the most frequently reported side effect is local, i.e. oral/sublingual itching (sometimes followed by gastrointestinal complaints such as stomach ache or nausea). These phenomena are always described as mild and self-resolving and only rarely did they lead to the discontinuation of the treatment. The occurrence rate of systemic side effects (asthma, urticaria/angioedema, rhinitis) in the actively treated patients was indeed very low and not significantly different from the corresponding placebo-treated groups. Noticeably, no severe systemic adverse event (near-fatal, grade IV) has ever been reported in the literature over 15 years.

André et al. [36] recently reviewed the safety aspects of the controlled trials performed with the vaccines of a single manufacturer. Six hundred and ninety subjects were enrolled (347 active + 343 placebo), 218 of them children (103 active + 115 placebo). The large majority of events were mild. All events had similar incidence in active and placebo, with the exception of the oral and gastrointestinal side effects, which were more frequent in SLIT patients, although they were always mild. The occurrence of side effects and dropouts was similar in adults and children.

Similarly, in the more recent pediatric studies, the occurrence of side effects was negligible and not worrying [18, 21, 28–31, 33]. In one study [28] a particularly high occurrence of gastrointestinal complaints was noted, but in this study the amount of allergen was very high: about 375 times the amount usually administered in a standard subcutaneous course.

Comparison of SLIT and SCIT

As far as the direct comparison between SLIT and SCIT is concerned there is a single double-blind double-dummy study published as a full paper [37]. It showed that SLIT had a clinical efficacy superimposable to SCIT (symptoms and need for drugs), but that SLIT was better accepted and tolerated by the patients. Another well-designed rigorous double-dummy trial with birch pollen extract has recently been published in abstract form [38]. The study showed that SLIT and injection IT had a similar efficacy, but only with SCIT did systemic side effects of grade III and IV appear, whereas SLIT was comparable to placebo.

As mentioned before, no near fatal or severe systemic event has ever been reported with SLIT. On the other hand, if we look at the recent literature, the rate of occurrence of severe systemic (near-fatal) adverse events with SCIT ranges between 0.5 and 6% [39, 40]. Concerning the rate of occurrence of systemic reactions in general, a comprehensive review by Stewart and Lockey [41] on SCIT reported the following figures: (1) 0.8–46.7% with conventional schedules, (2) 0–16.7% with modified allergens, and (3) 0–21% with accelerated or rush schedules. These are on average higher than those reported with SLIT. As a general consideration it is surprising that in about 20% of the published studies with SCIT there is no information at all concerning side effects, and in the remaining studies side effects are reported only in an incomplete manner [42], with an average occurrence of systemic effects in 24% of the patients. No fatality has ever been reported with SLIT, which is at variance with SCIT, where more than 50 cases are well documented [for review, see 43].

Finally, no experimental data are available on the compliance with SLIT. On the other hand, the few trials [44, 45] investigating the compliance with SCIT evidenced that the rate of discontinuation of the treatment ranged between 10 and 34% [44] and that up to 50% of the patients were noncompliant because of the occurrence of intolerable side effects [45].

Experimental Evidence: Safety of SLIT in the Postmarketing Surveillance Studies

The information on safety provided by the controlled trials are of course valuable, but the populations are highly selected and the administration of SLIT is usually supervised: this situation is profoundly different from that occurring in the clinical reality. Therefore, more consistent information on the safety should be obtained when SLIT is prescribed and administered in the everyday clinical practice, i.e. in postmarketing surveillance studies.

An early study of pharmacovigilance [46] reported that the incidence of side effects was indeed low: oropharyngeal itching represented about 50% of the untoward effects, followed by rhinorrhea and constipation. Urticaria and asthma were very rare. More than 90% of the effects were mild and did not require any kind of medical treatment. No systemic anaphylaxis was reported.

A pharmacosurveillance study performed in 268 children aged between 2 and 15 years and having received SLIT for up to 3 years showed that the overall incidence of systemic side effects involved 3% of the patients and 1/12,000 doses. Out of 8 side effects, only one (urticaria) was moderate and required treatment with a single dose of oral antihistamine. Overall, in none of the patients was the treatment discontinued [47].

Another pharmacosurveillance study in adult patients was recently published [48]. One hundred and ninety-eight patients were observed while receiving SLIT either preseasonally or continuously over a 3-year period. Side effects were observed in 7.5% of patients and 0.52/1,000 doses administered. Four urticaria and 2 gastrointestinal complaints were judged as moderate. Also in this study, side effects were controlled by a temporary dose adjustment and in no case was the treatment discontinued.

SLIT and the Oral Mucosa

It has sometimes been claimed that SLIT can lead to an increased risk in patients suffering from the oral allergy syndrome. The sublingual administration of pollen allergens which are cross-reacting with food allergens may in fact elicit local edema and swelling. Indeed, a controlled study (30 subjects) performed in patients with a certain oral allergy syndrome, receiving an allergoid in orosoluble tablets did not confirm this hypothesis [49].

In another clinical trial, the possible immunological effects of the sublingual administration of allergens were investigated by measuring the mucosal level of tryptase and ECP. These mediators are markers of mast cell degranulation and eosinophil activation, respectively. No change in the levels of these mediators could be detected at all, even in one patient reporting oral itching after SLIT intake [50].

One of the earliest concerns about the safety of SLIT was the envisaged possibility of a too rapid absorption of the allergen through oral mucosa [10]. Indeed, pharmacokinetics studies, performed in healthy and allergic volunteers using a radiolabeled allergen, showed that no sublingual absorption occurs until the allergen is kept under the tongue without swallowing [51, 52]. The absorption seems to begin after the allergen has reached the gastrointestinal tract. On the other hand, a long-lasting persistence of the radiolabeled allergen, adsorbed to the oral mucosa, could be detected.

Safety of LNIT

Fourteen randomized controlled clinical trials with LNIT are at present available [for review, see 12]. Thirteen out of the 14 papers demonstrate a significant improvement of nasal symptoms both in perennial and seasonal rhinitis; two studies were conducted in children. The effects of LNIT seem to be restricted to the target organ only; its effectiveness is dose-related and, at least for pollen allergy, a preseasonal course should be repeated every year [53]. Concerning the safety, it can be seen that the earliest aqueous extracts, although effective, were associated with troublesome local side effects, i.e. mild rhinitis symptoms. The usefulness of LNIT became, therefore, somewhere questionable [54]. On the other hand, the modified extracts showed a lower incidence of side effects, but they also appeared to be less effective. Recently, micronized dried-powder preparations have been manufactured and commercialized. These extracts show an efficacy comparable to that of the aqueous ones and appear almost completely devoid of local side effects [55]. This is probably due to a better titration of the build-up phase doses. The hypothesized risk of an induction of an asthma attack is not substantiated by the evidence: such an event has only been described anedoctally in 3 patients in a single study [56], probably due to the wrong technique of administration. Moreover, some manufacturers suggest a nasal premedication with cromolyn, which contributes to reducing the nasal side effects.

Also in the case of nasal IT, no direct absorption through the nasal mucosa could be detected [52]. The allergen sprayed into the nose is slowly transported towards the pharynx by the mucociliary clearance and then swallowed, although a relevant fraction persists on the nasal mucosa for hours.

As mentioned before, LNIT requires a particular administration technique: after premedication, the allergenic extract (aqueous or powdered) has to be sprayed into a nostril while vocalizing. This fact, in addition to the efficacy limited to the nose, reduced the clinical use of LNIT; therefore, no postmarketing surveillance studies are available. In conclusion, based on the clinical trials, LNIT appears safe and well tolerated. The EAACI/ESPACI position paper states that 'side effects do not represent a problem' [12].

Conclusions

The results from the randomized controlled clinical trials are overall favorable and justify the recent official approval of SLIT for the routine clinical use in children and adults [13]. The safety profile, as derived from both controlled trials and postmarketing surveys, is extremely favorable, especially when compared to SCIT. In fact, looking at the figures from the literature, the rate of systemic adverse events, in particular severe ones, is clearly higher with the subcutaneous administration. The most frequent side effects seen with SLIT are local ones (sublingual itching) followed by gastrointestinal complaints (stomach ache and/or nausea). Nevertheless, these effects virtually never lead to a discontinuation of the treatment; they are mild and self-resolving and can be easily controlled by a temporary dose reduction. In general, the risk/benefit ratio of SLIT seems to be favorable.

Although the safety profile of SLIT is satisfactory, it is important to underline that physicians who prescribe IT need adequate training in allergology and specialist supervision is always necessary. The therapy should only be prescribed by specialists, after a detailed diagnosis has been made and the expected benefit/cost ratio has been carefully evaluated. Patients should be instructed to carefully follow the manufacturer's schedule of administration and to visit the clinic at least every 3 months. Only standardized extracts with proven efficacy (grass, *Parietaria*, mites, olive, birch) should be used. Since SLIT (and LNIT) is self-administered, detailed instructions and follow-up of the patients are mandatory.

Clinical studies have only been conducted for 15 years, and therefore several points still need to be clarified [57]. One of the most important points is the optimal dose of allergen to be administered: it is known that the use of very high amounts of allergen is associated with gastrointestinal symptoms, whereas too low doses are ineffective (fig. 1). Based on the available data, an effective and safe dose should be between about 20 and 300 times higher than

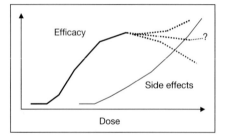

Fig. 1. Hypothesis on the relationship among dose, efficacy and side effects. It is not clear whether increasing the doses leads to a better efficacy, but it is ascertained that side effects become more frequent.

for the subcutaneous route, but this interval is wide and there are no dose-ranging studies.

The sublingual route appears particularly suitable for pediatric patients, because it is well accepted and safe. Therefore, SLIT represents a significant step towards an optimal allergy management.

References

1 Noon L: Prophylactic inoculation against hay fever. Lancet 1911;i:1572–1573.
2 Black JH: The oral administration of pollen: Clinical report. J Lab Clin Med 1928;13:709.
3 Dunbar P: The present state of knowledge of hayfever. J Hyg 1913;13:105.
4 Passalacqua G, Albano M, Riccio A, et al: Local nasal immunotherapy: Experimental evidences and general considerations. Allergy 1997;52(33 suppl):10–16.
5 Herxeimer H: Bronchial hypersensitization and hyposensitization in man. Int Arch Allergy Appl Immunol 1951;40:40–57.
6 Committee on the Safety of Medicines. CSM update. Desensitizing vaccines. Br Med J 1986; 293:948.
7 Lockey RF, Benedict LM, Turkeltaub PC, Bukantz SC: Fatalities from immunotherapy and skin testing. J Allergy Clin Immunol 1987;79:660–677.
8 Reid MJ, Lockey RF, Turkeltaub PC, Platt-Mills TAE: Survey of fatalities from skin testing and immunotherapy. J Allergy Clin Immunol 1993;92:6–15.
9 Rogala B: Risk and safety of specific immunotherapy. Allergy 1998;53:473–477.
10 Malling HJ, Weeke B: EAACI immunotherapy position paper. Allergy 1993;48(suppl 14):9–35.
11 World Health Organization Position Paper: Allergen immunotherapy: Therapeutical vaccines for allergic diseases. Allergy 1998;53(suppl 44):20–22.
12 Malling HJ: EAACI position paper on local immunotherapy. Allergy 1998;53:933–944.
13 ARIA: Allergic rhinitis and its impact on asthma. Position paper endorsed by WHO. J Allergy Clin Immunol 2001;108(suppl):240–245.
14 Tari MG, Mancino M, Monti G: Efficacy of sublingual immunotherapy in patients with rhinitis and asthma due to house dust mite. A double blind study. Allergol Immunopathol 1990;18:277–284.
15 Sabbah A, Hassoun S, Le Sellin J, Andre C, Sicard H: A double blind placebo controlled trial by the sublingual route of immunotherapy with a standardized grass pollen extract. Allergy 1994;49: 309–313.
16 Troise C, Voltolini S, Canessa A, Pecora S, Negrini AC: Sublingual immunotherapy in Parietaria pollen-induced rhinitis: A double blind study. J Investig Allergol Clin Immunol 1995;5:25–30.
17 Feliziani V, Lattuada G, Parmiani S, Dall'Aglio PP: Safety and efficacy of sublingual rush immunotherapy with grass allergen extracts. A double blind study. Allergol Immunopathol 1995; 23:173–178.

18   Hirsch T, Sahn M, Leupold W: Double blind placebo controlled study of sublingual immuno-therapy with house dust mite extracts in children. Pediatr Allergy Immunol 1997;8:21–27.

19   Clavel R, Bousquet J, André C: Clinical efficacy of sublingual swallow immunotherapy: A double blind placebo controlled trial of a standardized five grass pollen extract in rhinitis. Allergy 1998; 53:493–498.

20   Horak F, Stubner UE, Berger U, Marks B, Toth J, Jager S: Immunotherapy with sublingual birch pollen extract: A short-term double-blind study. J Investig Allergol Clin Immunol 1998;8: 165–171.

21   Vourdas D, Syrigou E, Potamianou P, et al: Double-blind placebo-controlled evaluation of sublingual immunotherapy with a standardized olive tree pollen extract in pediatric patients with allergic rhinoconjunctivitis and mild asthma due to olive tree pollen sensitization. Allergy 1998; 53:662–671.

22   Hordijk GJ, Antwelink JB, Luwema RA: Sublingual immunotherapy with a standardized grass pollen extract: A double-blind placebo-controlled study. Allergol Immunopathol 1998;26:234–240.

23   Passalacqua G, Albano M, Fregonese L, et al: Randomised controlled trial of local allergoid immunotherapy on allergic inflammation in mite induced rhinoconjunctivitis. Lancet 1998;351: 629–632.

24   Passalacqua G, Albano M, Riccio AM, et al: Clinical and immunological effects of a rush sub-lingual immunotherapy to Parietaria species: A double-blind placebo-controlled trial. J Allergy Clin Immunol 1999;104:964–968.

25   Bousquet J, Scheinmann P, Guinnepain MT, et al: Sublingual swallow immunotherapy (SLIT) in patients with asthma due to house dust mites: A double-blind placebo-controlled study. Allergy 1999;54:249–260.

26   Purello D'Ambrosio F, Gangemi S, Isola S, et al: Sublingual immunotherapy: A double-blind placebo-controlled trial with *Parietaria judaica* extract standardized in mass units in patients with rhinoconjunctivitis, asthma or both. Allergy 1999;54:968–973.

27   Pradalier A, Basset D, Claudel A, et al: Sublingual swallow immunotherapy (SLIT) with a standardized five grass pollen extract (drops and sublingual tablets) versus placebo in seasonal rhinitis. Allergy 1999;54:819–828.

28   La Rosa M, Ranno C, André C, Carat F, Tosca MA, Canonica GW: Double-blind placebo-controlled evaluation of sublingual swallow immunotherapy with standardized *Parietaria judaica* extract in children with allergic rhinoconjunctivitis. J Allergy Clin Immunol 1999;104:425–432.

29   Guez S, Vatrinet C, Fadel R, André C: House dust mite sublingual swallow immunotherapy in perennial rhinitis: A double-blind placebo-controlled study. Allergy 2000;55:369–375.

30   Pajno GB, Morabito L, Barberio G, Parmiani S: Clinical and immunological effects of long-term sublingual immunotherapy in asthmatic children sensitized to mite: A double-blind study. Allergy 2000;55:842–849.

31   Caffarelli C, Sensi LG, Marcucci F, Cavagni C: Preseasonal local allergoid immunotherapy to grass pollen in children: A double-blind, placebo-controlled, randomized trial. Allergy 2000;55: 1142–1147.

32   Ariano R, Spadolini I, Panzani RC: Efficacy of sublingual specific immunotherapy in Cupressaceae allergy using an extract of *Cupressus arizonica*. A double-blind study. Allergol Immunopathol (Madr) 2001;29:238–244.

33   Bahceciler NN, Isik U, Barlan IB, Basaran N: Efficacy of sublingual immunotherapy in children with asthma and rhinitis: A double-blind, placebo-controlled study. Pediatr Pulmonol 2001;32: 49–55.

34   Voltolini S, Modena P, Minale P, et al: Sublingual immunotherapy in tree pollen allergy. Double-blind, placebo-controlled study with a biologically standardized extract of tree pollen (alder, birch and hazel) administered by a rush schedule. Allergol Immunopathol (Madr) 2001;29:103–110.

35   Lima MT, Watson D, Pitkin L, et al: Grass pollen sublingual immunotherapy for seasonal rhinoconjunctivitis: A randomized controlled trial. Clin Exp Allergy 2002;32:507–514.

36   André C, Vatrinet C, Galvain S, Carat F, Sicard H: Safety of sublingual swallow immunotherapy in children and adults. Int Arch Allergy Immunol 2000;121:229–234.

37   Quirino T, Iemoli E, Siciliani E, Parmiani S: Sublingual vs injective immunotherapy in grass pollen allergic patients: A double-blind double-dummy study. Clin Exp Allergy 1996;26: 1253–1261.

38 Khinchi S, Poulsen LK, Carat F, André C, Malling HJ: Clinical efficacy of sublingual swallow and subcutaneous immunotherapy in patients with allergic rhinoconjunctivitis due to birch pollen. A double-blind double-dummy placebo-controlled study. 19th EAACI Congress, Lisbon (abstract). Allergy 2000;55(suppl 63):24.

39 Tinkelman DG, Cole WQ, Tunno J: Immunotherapy: A one-year prospective study to evaluate risk factors of systemic reactions. J Allergy Clin Immunol 1995;95:8–14.

40 Ostergaard PA, Kaad PH, Kristensen T: A prospective study on the safety of immunotherapy in children with severe asthma. Allergy 1986;41:588–593.

41 Stewart GE, Lockey RF: Systemic reactions from allergen immunotherapy. J Allergy Clin Immunol 1992;90:567–578.

42 Malling HJ: Immunotherapy as an effective tool in allergy treatment. Allergy 1998;53:461–472.

43 Lockey RF, Nicoara Kasti GL, Theodoropoulos DS, Bukantz SC: Systemic reactions and fatalities associated with allergen immunotherapy. Ann Allergy Asthma Immunol 2001;87(suppl 1): 47–55.

44 Lower T, Hensy J, Mandik L, et al: Compliance with allergen immunotherapy. Ann Allergy 1993; 70:480–482.

45 Cohn JR, Pizzi A: Determinants of patient compliance with allergen immunotherapy. J Allergy Clin Immunol 1993;91:734–737.

46 Almangro E, Assensio O, Bartolomé JM, et al: Estudio multicentrico de farmacovigilancia de imunoterapia sublingual en pacientes alergicos. Allergol Immunopathol 1995;23:153.

47 Di Rienzo V, Pagani A, Parmiani S, Passalacqua G, Canonica GW: Post-marketing surveillance study on the safety of sublingual immunotherapy in children. Allergy 1999;54:1110–1113.

48 Lombardi C, Gargioni S, Melchiorre A, Tiri A, Falagiani P, Canonica GW, Passalacqua G: Safety of sublingual immunotherapy in adults: A post-marketing surveillance study. Allergy 2001;56: 889–892.

49 Lombardi C, Canonica GW, Passalacqua G: Sublingual immunotherapy is clinically safe in patients with oral allergy syndrome. Allergy 2000;55:677–678.

50 Frati F, Marcucci F, Sensi L, Passalacqua G: Sublingual tryptase and ECP in children treated with grass pollen sublingual immunotherapy: Safety and immunological implications. Allergy 2001; 56:1091–1095.

51 Bagnasco M, Passalacqua G, Villa G, et al: Pharmacokinetics of an allergen and a monomeric allergoid for oromucosal immunotherapy in allergic volunteers. Clin Exp Allergy 2001;31:54–60.

52 Bagnasco M, Mariani G, Passalacqua G, et al: Absorption and distribution kinetics of the major Parietaria allergen (Par j 1) administered by noninjectable routes to healthy human beings. J Allergy Clin Immunol 1997;100:122–129.

53 Passalacqua G, Albano M, Pronzato C, Riccio A, Falagiani P, Canonica GW: Long-term follow-up of nasal immunotherapy to Parietaria: Clinical and immunological effects. Clin Exp Allergy 1997;27:904–908.

54 Bjorksten B: Local immunotherapy is not documented for clinical use. Allergy 1994;49:299–301.

55 Passalacqua G, Bagnasco M, Mariani G, Falagiani P, Canonica GW: Local immunotherapy: Pharmacokinetics and efficacy. Allergy 1998;53:477–484.

56 D'Amato G, Lobefalo G, Liccardi G, Cazzola M: A double-blind placebo-controlled trial of local nasal immunotherapy in allergic rhinitis to Parietaria pollen. Clin Exp Allergy 1995;25:141–148.

57 Frew AJ, Smith PJ: Sublingual immunotherapy. J Allergy Clin Immunol 2001;107:441–444.

Giovanni Passalacqua, MD
Allergy and Respiratory Diseases, DIMI, Genoa University,
Padiglione Maragliano, L.go R. Benzi 10, I–16132 Genoa (Italy)
Tel. +39 10 3538908, Fax +39 10 3538904
E-Mail giovanni.passalacqua@hsanmartino.liguria.it

Markert UR, Elsner P (eds): Local Immunotherapy in Allergy.
Chem Immunol Allergy. Basel, Karger, 2003, vol 82, pp 119–126

·······················

The WHO ARIA (Allergic Rhinitis and Its Impact on Asthma) Initiative

C. Bachert, P. van Cauwenberge

Department of Oto-Rhino-Laryngology, Ghent University Hospital, Ghent, Belgium

Key Words
Rhinitis · Asthma · Immunotherapy, specific

Abstract
The ARIA working group, in collaboration with the WHO in Geneva, recently published a state-of-the-art review and recommendations derived from it on the link between rhinitis and asthma. Rhinitis is the most frequent manifestation of allergic disease in humans and is often linked to other atopic diseases such as food allergy, atopic dermatitis or asthma, and may furthermore have an impact on the sinuses. ARIA focuses on one of the most important of the mentioned issues, the link between upper and lower airways in allergic disease. To facilitate understanding between the otorhinolaryngologist and the pulmonologist, the classification of rhinitis has been adapted to that of asthma, and the terms 'intermittent' and 'persistent' allergic rhinitis have been introduced. Elaborate guidelines for the diagnosis and assessment of the severity of disease are provided, and detailed recommendations for the management of rhinitis and asthma are suggested with a special focus on specific immunotherapy.

The ARIA paper [1] summarizes current knowledge on rhinitis and its link to asthma and features several main issues, presenting a new classification of rhinitis with reference to a similar classification as is currently used for asthma. Because of the long-term exposure to seasonal allergens in some countries and the seasonal variations also observed in mite allergen exposure [2], it was decided that the terms 'seasonal' and 'perennial' would not be very helpful for any decision in terms of treatment. Furthermore, seasonal and perennial

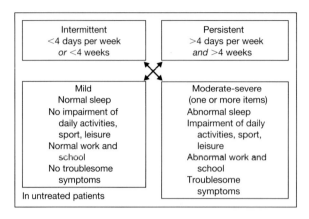

Intermittent <4 days per week *or* <4 weeks	Persistent >4 days per week *and* >4 weeks
Mild Normal sleep No impairment of daily activities, sport, leisure Normal work and school No troublesome symptoms In untreated patients	Moderate-severe (one or more items) Abnormal sleep Impairment of daily activities, sport, leisure Abnormal work and school Troublesome symptoms

Fig. 1. Classification of allergic rhinitis according to the WHO ARIA work group.

allergens may considerably differ from one place to another, so that the offending allergen has to be mentioned separately. It was therefore decided to use the terms 'intermittent' and 'persistent' allergic rhinitis. Persistent allergic rhinitis means more than 4 days of symptoms per week and more than 4 weeks of symptoms, and may be either seen during the season or due to an allergen exposure during the year. In contrast, intermittent means less than 4 days per week or less than 4 weeks of symptoms, which again may be based on seasonal or perennial allergens. The term persistent also reflects the concept of minimal persistent inflammation, which has been described for the nasal mucosa as an ongoing inflammation even without acute symptoms [3]. It is estimated that about two thirds of the patients suffer from intermittent and one third from persistent rhinitis, and that this terminology is independent from seasonal or perennial allergic rhinitis. The severity of disease was furthermore classified as mild or moderate to severe, depending on the symptoms, but also on the impact of those symptoms on quality of life issues such as sleep, impairment of daily activities and work performance (fig. 1).

The large body of epidemiological studies have clearly shown that allergic rhinitis and asthma are frequent diseases, and that both diseases obviously still increase in prevalence [4, 5]. However, without any doubt, there is a direct link between rhinitis and asthma. Several studies in a large number of patients have clearly shown that rhinitis sufferers have a 3- to 7-fold increased risk to also develop asthma within 7 years compared to normal controls. Most of this development actually lies in the early years of childhood, as was recently shown in the MAS and PAT studies [6, 7]. In the first study, 5-year-old children sensitized to pollen with allergic rhinitis symptoms developed asthma within 2 years in 34%, and in the second study, children 6–14 years of age with pollen-allergic rhinitis developed asthma within three seasons in 44%. Furthermore, 20% of children without a history of asthma developed asthma symptoms within the first season, so that it can be estimated that at least 35% of children of this age develop asthmatic symptoms within just two seasons. This natural development of atopic disease clearly asks for intervention in terms of the prevention of disease expansion.

The WHO initiative ARIA [1] therefore formulated a number of recommendations, which are listed below:

(1) Allergic rhinitis is a major chronic respiratory disease because of its prevalence, its impact on the quality of life, its impact on work/school performance and productivity, its economic burden, and its links with asthma.

(2) In addition, allergic rhinitis is associated with sinusitis and other comorbidities such as conjunctivitis.

(3) It is recommended that allergic rhinitis should be considered as a risk factor for asthma along with other known risk factors.

(4) A new subdivision of allergic rhinitis has been proposed: intermittent and persistent.

(5) The severity of allergic rhinitis has been classified as 'mild' and 'moderate/severe' depending on the severity of symptoms and quality of life outcomes.

(6) Depending on the subdivision and severity of allergic rhinitis, a stepwise therapeutic approach has been proposed.

(7) The treatment of allergic rhinitis combines: allergen avoidance (when possible), pharmacotherapy and immunotherapy.

(8) It is recommended that patients with persistent allergic rhinitis be evaluated for asthma by history, chest examination and, if possible and when necessary, assessment of airflow obstruction before and after bronchodilator.

(9) It is recommended that history and examination of the upper respiratory tract for allergic rhinitis are performed in patients with asthma.

(10) It is recommended to propose a strategy combining the treatment of both the upper and lower airway disease in terms of efficacy and safety.

Although we do not fully understand the pathomechanisms behind this relationship, several possibilities have been proposed, such as the nasal-bronchial reflex, aspiration of nasal contents, the effect of mouth breathing and the release of mediators due to allergen exposure in the nose. Of these, the hypothesis of a signal released at the side of exposure to the bone marrow with consecutive mobilization of inflammatory progenitor cells is currently favored (fig. 2). Several studies have contributed to this hypothesis, which is primarily based on observations in dogs, but recently has also got more and more support in humans [8]. Chakir et al. [9], for example, showed that the number of T cells

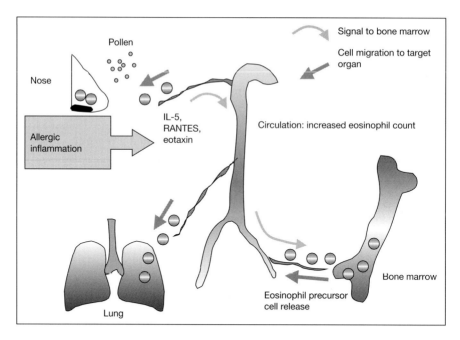

Fig. 2. Current concept of nose-lung interactions via signals to the bone marrow.

and eosinophils in bronchial biopsies increased in patients with seasonal allergic rhinitis symptoms only. This would indicate that, although not symptomatic, there is an ongoing minimal inflammation in the lower airways in patients with allergic rhinitis. This inflammation can lead to a clear late-phase response in the lower airways, which is seen not only in patients with allergic asthma, but also in patients with allergic rhinitis only [10]. Whenever an allergen would reach the lower airways, it could induce a typical allergic inflammatory reaction. Finally, Braunstahl et al. [11] recently showed that not only allergen exposure of the nose would cause bronchial inflammation, but also allergen exposure of the bronchi would induce an increase in inflammatory cells in the nasal mucosa. A possible candidate to transfer this signal to the bone marrow is interleukin-5, but also chemokines, specifically for eosinophils, could well be involved. These data support the clinical observation of a strong link between the lower and upper airways and help us to understand the basic pathomechanisms behind it.

After elaborate guidelines for the diagnosis and assessment of the severity of disease, which will not be covered in this summary, the ARIA report also gives detailed recommendations for the management of rhinitis and to some extent asthma, which in contrast to former reports are evidence-based. The paper

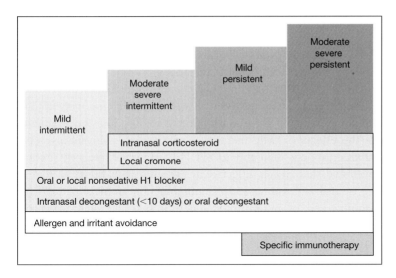

Fig. 3. Stepwise approach to the treatment of allergic rhinitis.

proposes a stepwise approach to a therapy consisting of allergen avoidance, drug treatment and specific immunotherapy (SIT) (fig. 3). Here, we focus on the role of SIT in this treatment concept.

SIT is the standard of care for hymenopterous sting-induced systemic allergic reactions and has clearly been shown to be also effective for the treatment of seasonal and perennial allergic rhinoconjunctivitis and asthma [12]. It has been shown that SIT can interfere with basic pathophysiological mechanisms of allergic disease and may be able to prevent the development of asthma in patients with allergic rhinitis. Thus, SIT is recommended as a supplement to allergen avoidance and drug therapy to make the patient as symptom-free as possible, but should also be initiated early in the disease process to prevent further development of severe disease and to reduce the risk of side effects. According to the recommendations, subcutaneous SIT is the standard procedure; local SIT (nasal or sublingual-swallow immunotherapy) may be considered in selected patients with systemic side effects and who refuse injection treatment.

The indications for SIT are given below:

(1) Carefully selected patients with rhinitis, conjunctivitis and/or asthma caused by pollen, house dust mite or cat allergy. Immunotherapy is also indicated when asthma during the pollen season complicates rhinoconjunctivitis.

(2) When H1 antihistamines and intranasal pharmacotherapy insufficiently control symptoms or produce undesirable side effects.

(3) When patients do not want to receive long-term pharmacotherapy for their treatment.

The efficacy of subcutaneous SIT has been clearly shown in a meta-analysis of 43 double-blind placebo-controlled trials in allergic rhinitis as well as another meta-analysis of 16 double-blind placebo-controlled studies in asthma patients [13]. The mean clinical improvement was 45% reduction in symptoms and medication compared with placebo in rhinitis and 40% in asthma patients, which exceeds the effects of drug therapy. A recent meta-analysis also confirmed that asthma responds favorably to SIT [14]. However, recently it could also be demonstrated that SIT is effective in patients with house dust mite allergy, allergic rhinitis and asthma [15]. Immunotherapy in these patients not only reduced rhinitis and asthma symptoms as well as rescue medication, but also had an impact on bronchial hyperreactivity over the 3-year follow-up period.

It is of special interest that SIT has been shown to prevent new sensitizations in controlled studies [16] and also in large open observational studies [17]. In the first study, SIT was applied in children monosensitized to house dust mite over a 3-year period. In the SIT group, about half of the patients developed new sensitizations, whereas in the control group, all the subjects developed new sensitizations to perennial and seasonal allergens during the follow-up period. In the second study, looking at a group of more than 7,000 patients with immunotherapy compared to more than 1,000 patients with drug therapy, about 30% of the SIT group was polysensitized after 7 years, whereas nearly 80% of the drug group showed polysensitizations after this period. In this latter group, there was also a significant increase in total IgE mean values versus the SIT-treated group. Thus, SIT is able to prevent new sensitizations in allergic rhinitis subjects.

However, the question of whether SIT could actually prevent the development of asthma in children with rhinitis was answered only recently. In a study in children aged 6–14 years with birch or timothy pollen-allergic rhinitis, who had followed immunotherapy for 3 years, there was a significant reduction of conjunctivitis and rhinitis symptoms in the SIT group, a significant reduction in conjunctival sensitivity and also an improvement of bronchial hyperreactivity [7]. Furthermore, significantly fewer children in the SIT group developed asthma in three seasons compared to the control group, with an odds ratio of 2.5.

In conclusion, the ARIA WHO workgroup emphasized the link between rhinitis and asthma and declared rhinitis a major chronic respiratory disease and a risk factor for the development of lower airway disease. It is therefore critical to treat both airway manifestations in a combined strategy, and immunotherapy has been proven to be a suitable treatment when patients are selected carefully.

It must be our aim to prevent the development of asthma in patients, especially in children with rhinitis, and SIT has been shown to considerably reduce the risk of disease expansion in this group of patients that otherwise would develop asthma in about 35–45% of cases. SIT clearly is a treatment of choice for common airway disease such as a reductive and preventive treatment approach. Further studies are needed to confirm this benefit and to allow a better classification of patients suitable for preventive SIT in terms of sensitizations, age and laboratory parameters.

References

1 Bousquet J, Van Cauwenberge P, Khaltaev N: Allergic rhinitis and its impact on asthma. J Allergy Clin Immunol 2001;108:S147–S334.
2 Platts-Mills TA, Thomas WR, Aalberse RC, Vervloet D, Champman MD: Dust mite allergens and asthma: Report of a second international workshop. J Allergy Clin Immunol 1992;89:1046–1060.
3 Ciprandi G, Buscaglia S, Pesce G, et al: Minimal persistent inflammation is present at mucosal level in patients with asymptomatic rhinitis and mite allergy. J Allergy Clin Immunol 1995;96: 971–979.
4 Wuthrich B, Schindler C, Leuenberger P, Ackermann-Liebrich U: Prevalence of atopy and pollinosis in the adult population of Switzerland (SAPALDIA study). Swiss Study on Air Pollution and Lung Diseases in Adults. Int Arch Allergy Immunol 1995;106:149–156.
5 Asher MI, Keil U, Anderson HR, et al: International Study of Asthma and Allergies in Childhood (ISAAC): Rationale and methods. Eur Respir J 1995;8:483–491.
6 Wahn U, Bergmann R, Kulig M, Forster J, Bauer CP: The natural course of sensitisation and atopic disease in infancy and childhood. Pediatr Allergy Immunol 1997;8:16–20.
7 Moller C, Dreborg S, Ferdousi HA, Halken S, Host A, Jacobsen L, Koivikko A, Koller DY, Niggemann B, Norberg LA, Urbanek R, Valovirta E, Wahn U: Pollen immunotherapy reduces the development of asthma in children with seasonal rhinoconjunctivitis (the PAT study). J Allergy Clin Immunol 2002;109:251–256.
8 Denburg JA, Sehmi R, Saito H, Pil-Seob J, Inman MD, O'Byrne PM: Systemic aspects of allergic disease: Bone marrow responses. J Allergy Clin Immunol 2000;106:S242–S246.
9 Chakir J, Laviolette M, Boutet M, Laliberte R, Dube J, Boulet LP: Lower airways remodeling in nonasthmatic subjects with allergic rhinitis. Lab Invest 1996;75:735–744.
10 Alvarez MJ, Olaguibel JM, Garcia BE, Tabar AI, Urbiola E: Comparison of allergen-induced changes in bronchial hyperresponsiveness and airway inflammation between mildly allergic asthma patients and allergic rhinitis patients. Allergy 2000;55:531–539.
11 Braunstahl GJ, Kleinjan A, Overbeek SE, Prins JB, Hoogsteden HC, Fokkens WJ: Segmental bronchial provocation induces nasal inflammation in allergic rhinitis patients. Am J Respir Crit Care Med 2000;161:2051–2057.
12 Bousquet J, Lockey R, Malling H: Allergen immunotherapy: Therapeutic vaccines for allergic diseases. WHO position paper. J Allergy Clin Immunol 1998;102:558–562.
13 Abramson MJ, Puy RM, Weiner JM: Allergen immunotherapy for asthma. Cochrane Database Syst Rev 2000;CD001186.
14 Malling H: Immunotherapy. Position paper of the EAACI. Allergy 1988;43(suppl 6):228–238.
15 Pichler CE, Helbling A, Pichler WJ: Three years of specific immunotherapy with house-dust-mite extracts in patients with rhinitis and asthma: Significant improvement of allergen-specific parameters and of nonspecific bronchial hyperreactivity. Allergy 2001;56:301–306.
16 Des Roches A, Paradis L, Knani J, et al: Immunotherapy with a standardized *Dermatophagoides pteronyssinus* extract. Duration of efficacy of immunotherapy after its cessation. Allergy 1996;51: 430–433.

17   Purello-D'Ambrosio F, Gangemi S, Merendino RA, Isola S, Puccinelli P, Parmiani S, Ricciardi L:
     Prevention of new sensitizations in monosensitized subjects submitted to specific immunotherapy
     or not. A retrospective study. Clin Exp Allergy 2001;31:1295–1302.

Professor Claus Bachert, MD, PhD
Department of Oto-Rhino-Laryngology,
Ghent University Hospital,
B–9000 Ghent (Belgium)
Tel. +32 9240 2363, Fax +32 9240 4993, E-Mail claus.bachert@rug.ac.be

Markert UR, Elsner P (eds): Local Immunotherapy in Allergy.
Chem Immunol Allergy. Basel, Karger, 2003, vol 82, pp 127–135

....

Local Immunotherapy in Allergy: Prospects for the Future

Udo R. Markert

Department of Dermatology and Allergology and Department of Obstetrics,
Friedrich Schiller University, Jena, Germany

Key Words
Sublingual immunotherapy · Nasal immunotherapy · Allergy

Abstract
Sublingual immunotherapy in allergy is a promising method invented in its preliminary form almost 100 years ago, but applied in practice for only several years. A continuously increasing number of controlled studies indicate the efficacy of this method, but nevertheless numerous questions concerning immunological mechanisms, mode of application or long-term (side) effects remain to be answered and are responsible for keeping clinicians from pre-scribing it. Thus far, only a few studies compare the local and subcutaneous application of immunotherapy, but since the most efficient mode of application still remains far from being determined, such comparisons cannot be used for a general or definite recommendation of one of both therapies. The studies also fail to take into consideration patients' compliance or accept-ance of different types of therapies depending upon the previous duration and state of allergy. Although the acquiescence of local immunotherapies by physicians and patients is increasing, the topic will continue to offer material for years of emotional and scientific discussions.

Dosage

For all kinds of immunotherapy the question of dose is still discussed controversially. Is a single dose more relevant or a cumulative dose? The single and cumulative sublingual immunotherapy (SLIT) doses applied in published studies are from 5-fold up to several 100-fold higher than in subcutaneous immunotherapy [1]. Considering the possible mechanisms of immunotherapies, especially on the dendritic cell level, a balance of both might be expected to be the most convenient. All kinds of application produce a concentration gradient of allergens in the tissue. There are, whichever dose is given, dendritic cells receiving low amounts of allergens, but the number of affected cells and the highest concentrations of allergens absorbed by dendritic cells vary with increasing applied concentrations. Since the interleukin profile of dendritic cells depends upon the dose of allergens, the ratio of low-dose to high-dose stimulated cells might play a role in combination with the presence of additional tissue resident immune cells [2]. Their presence depends upon the duration and severity of the allergic disease, its localization as well as secondary or accompanying diseases or inflammations. Also substances therapeutically applied along with an allergen, as for example corticosteroids or mycophenolate mofetil, may be able to influence the function of dendritic cells or their interaction with T cells [3]. Since the underlying mechanisms are still widely unknown, convincing clinical recommendations require further investigations.

Intervals

The question of dosage is directly linked to the question of intervals. There are antigen-presenting cells homing, continuously entering and leaving the mucosa. Such cells are confronted with a high number of antigens and the medication represents only one out of many. Two things should be considered:(1) that other antigens present on the mucosa influence the effects of SLIT and (2) how many hours it takes to replace the leaving dendritic cells with native ones [4, 5]. Such a period of approximately 24 h might be a recommendable interval for SLIT applications, but it can only be speculated about this as long as more detailed studies are lacking [6].

Preparations and Application

Thus far, the best recommended application of SLIT is the swallow method [7]. It might be considered if other preparations, which provoke a longer allergen persistence on the mucosa, may be more effective or may at least reduce the necessary allergen concentration. Such preparations might be for example soluble tablets, which slowly dissolve in the mouth or chewing gum, which slowly releases the allergens [8–10]. It may also be taken into contemplation to add substances, which prolong the persistence of allergens on or increase their absorbance through the mucosa or which influence quantity and quality of saliva, especially in regard to immunoactive substances and enzymes [11, 12]. Dry preparations, such as tablets, have the advantage of requiring less or no conservation factors such as phenole, which might induce undesired effects in a few cases.

Adjuvant Therapies

As reflected in another chapter of this volume, especially anti-inflammatory treatment by antihistamines, antileukotrienes or corticoids might influence the success of immunotherapies, because it normalizes and standardizes the immunological base of treatment [13]. In severe cases a reduction of IgE levels by anti-IgE antibodies or even a slight general immunosuppressive treatment may also be considerable [14].

Duration of Therapy

This problem is also linked with the question of single and cumulative doses, which vary widely in different studies [15]. Should the cumulative dose be reached within a short period or may it be more effective if it is distributed for a longer time span? Should therapy be abolished when symptoms decreased or disappeared or should it also be continued during additional symptom-free seasons? The answers probably depend again upon several factors, such as the kind of allergens. Short-term therapies similar to subcutaneous rush therapies were tried out, but results are still very limited [16].

Initiation of Therapy

In the case slight allergies ARIA recommends symptomatic treatment [7]. On the other hand, the shorter the period of time during which the disease persists and the slighter the symptoms are, the higher the efficacy of immunotherapies seems to be. It will be necessary to study further whether local immunotherapies are able to prevent the risk of additional sensitizations and the aggravation of the state of disease, as is shown for subcutaneous immunotherapy [17]. Such considerations may influence the view on the onset of immunotherapies.

Continuation during the Season when Symptoms Occur

The doses of allergens naturally taken up during the season vary widely depending upon numerous circumstances which can or cannot be influenced. To provide a certain minimum dose for each day, the continuation of immunotherapies during the season is necessary. The question of the continuation of immunotherapy during the season is combined with the question of the application of additional symptomatic therapies during immunotherapy, which was done in most studies. The treatment and absence of symptoms during the season is an important factor for the patients' compliance.

Combination Therapies in Multiple Allergies

The maximal number of simultaneously treated allergies remains speculation. There are no studies as regards this number and the way of application. It is not clear yet, if different allergens should be applied as one single dose or alternately at different time points, which gave promising results in our clinical practice. In such cases, the dominance or uniformity of the single allergies as well as cross-reactions should be considered. Because of the high interindividual differences between all allergic patients, it will be hard to form comparable groups for comparative controlled studies to analyze the problem and to propose general recommendations.

Application of Allergoids

The application of allergoids is a promising idea to reduce side effects by the prevention of IgE binding to the full allergen, but the role of fragments other than the symptom-inducing epitope in sensitization and desensitization is still an open question. The first clinical observations on sublingual application are promising [8, 18, 19].

Prevention of New Sensitizations

Following recent studies relaying that an atopic ambiance induced by maternal factors can provoke a risk of atopic diseases in the child, it should be recognized that after birth preexisting atopic diseases present an enormous risk factor for additional sensitizations [20]. Immunotherapies are seen as a curative treatment, which reduces the severity of allergies or even cures them and thereby reduces the risk of new sensitizations. This has been well demonstrated for subcutaneous immunotherapies, but there are still no convincing results for SLIT [21, 22].

Long-Term Effects

As local immunotherapies have been used routinely only for the last decade, data on long-term effects are still rare [23]. To achieve a higher acceptance of SLIT by the clinicians, it is necessary to resolve this urgent question.

Application in Pregnancy or during Immunological Disorders

The lower number of side effects of local immunotherapies might suggest their use in pregnancy. Since the immunological effects of immunotherapies and the immunological changes during pregnancy are still under investigation, their interferences are also far from being understood. Application of immunotherapies in pregnancy should be handled with very strict caution until more scientific data is available, although several observations do not indicate contrary effects [24–26]. Similarly, the interferences of immunotherapies with immunological disorders, which may be provoked by immunological diseases (for example, autoimmune diseases, HIV) themselves or by indirect immunological influences as a consequence of other diseases, such as infections or tumors, are still widely unknown and will be hard to investigate because of the large variety of possible cases.

Limitations of Applicable Allergens

Depending upon the different regions, a large number of allergens have been used thus far for local immunotherapies. However, there is still a number of allergens, mainly food allergens, which have not yet been tested for this therapy.

Side Effects

As extensively reported in the other chapters, in millions of applications of local immunotherapies lethal side effects were not observed and severe side effects were extremely rare [27]. However, it should always be our aim to reduce even low numbers and not severe side effects. It might be important to scientifically analyze the correlation of mucosal injuries with the severity of side effects, which was observed in clinical practice.

Compliance

As in any other therapy, compliance is an important factor in order to obtain positive results. In some groups of patients, especially those with a high professional duty or any other rigid daily obligations, compliance might be better with local immunotherapy. In other groups, the subcutaneous application might lead to a higher compliance. In local immunotherapies, the patient's compliance also depends especially upon the physicians' compliance, which is necessary to guide and motivate the patient throughout the long period of therapy.

Thus far, no comparative studies on the compliance of the different forms of therapy are available. In SLIT, compliance was only compared between the active and the placebo groups, where it was similar [28].

Ethical Aspects

New therapies offer new chances, but also carry new risks. The risks include unknown efficacy and unknown side effects, whereas the chances include higher efficacy, lower side effects or easier applicability. The patient should be informed in detail about possible benefits, problems and open questions of different alternative therapies, and should be involved in the decision. Even such steps increase compliance and thereby success. An acceptable ethical aspect for the consideration of a therapy may be the mean state or severity of a disease, which is necessary to convince a patient of the need for such a therapy. This level might be lower for noninvasive immunotherapies than for invasive immunotherapies, and an earlier initiation of any kind of immunotherapy seems to lead to greater success. This hypothesis has yet to be proved by clinical investigations in allergy.

Comparative Studies with Other (Immuno)Therapies

Only a low number of comparative studies or observations of local and subcutaneous immunotherapies have been published thus far [29, 30]. All of these and future studies need to consider that the mode of application of local immunotherapy has not yet reached its final version and that, therefore, such comparisons cannot be generalized for all possible application methods and allergens. Thus, although when perfectly performed, actual or upcoming studies should only be evaluated as preliminary ones, as long as more detailed information regarding immunological mechanisms and effects as well as official recommendations concerning application modalities are not available. Additionally, as mentioned in another paper in this volume, data comparing immunotherapies with symptomatic therapies should also be available for the evaluation of immunotherapies [31].

Economic Aspects

Economic aspects of local and subcutaneous immunotherapies probably play a role in the selection of therapies, although they should not. Since respective health systems, costs of medication and costs of medical working hours in each country differ widely, such reflections are difficult to generalize in brief. Major aspects to contemplate are the higher cumulative and thereby more expensive doses in local immunotherapies on the one hand, but on the other hand the lower frequency of medical visits might be positive for health insurances (but also negative for the doctors' economy). Since the long-term efficacy of local immunotherapies is still unclear, costs for repeated or additional treatments are impossible to estimate. In summary, too many variables influence the economic question to provide a general statement in this framework.

Conclusion

A large network of factors may influence the possible effects of (local) immunotherapies. They include mainly dosage and application varieties or additional therapies. A high number of animal and clinical studies will be necessary to analyze the effects of individual factors in more detail. Evaluating any study, it must be considered that the change of only one factor may lead to another positive or negative result. Therefore, a much higher number of international, controlled studies are required to give further official recommendations on doses and application procedures. Only well-based recommendations will significantly increase the acceptance of local immunotherapies and reduce the emotional aspects of the discussion. This seems to be a challenging task to perform within a few, short years, but could also be perceived as a hopeful, long-term goal.

Acknowledgment

We thank Justine S. Fitzgerald for the corrections and suggestions concerning the English language.

References

1   Morris DL, Kroker GF, Sabnis VK, Morris MS: Local immunotherapy in allergy. Chem Immunol Allergy. Basel, Karger, 2003, vol 82, pp 1–10.
2   Kahler H, Stuwe H, Cromwell O, Fiebig H: Reactivity of T cells with grass pollen allergen extract and allergoid. Int Arch Allergy Immunol 1999;120:146–157.
3   Mehling A, Grabbe S, Voskort M, Schwarz T, Luger TA, Beissert S: Mycophenolate mofetil impairs the maturation and function of murine dendritic cells. J Immunol 2000;165: 2374–2381.
4   Gagliardi MC, Sallusto F, Marinaro M, Vendetti S, Riccomi A, De Magistris MT: Effects of the adjuvant cholera toxin on dendritic cells: Stimulatory and inhibitory signals that result in the amplification of immune responses. Int J Med Microbiol 2002;291:571–575.

5   Simmons CP, Ghaem-Magami M, Petrovska L, Lopes L, Chain BM, Williams NA, Dougan G: Immunomodulation using bacterial enterotoxins. Scand J Immunol 2001;53:218–226.

6   Eriksson K, Ahlfors E, George-Chandy A, Kaiserlian D, Czerkinsky C: Antigen presentation in the murine oral epithelium. Immunology 1996;88:147–152.

7   Bousquet J, Van Cauwenberge P, Khaltaev N: Allergic rhinitis and its impact on asthma. J Allergy Clin Immunol 2001;108:S147–S334.

8   Lombardi C, Gargioni S, Melchiorre A, Tiri A, Falagiani P, Canonica GW, Passalacqua G: Safety of sublingual immunotherapy with monomeric allergoid in adults: Multicenter post-marketing surveillance study. Allergy 2001;56:989–992.

9   Pradalier A, Basset D, Claudel A, Couturier P, Wessel F, Galvain S, Andre C: Sublingual-swallow immunotherapy (SLIT) with a standardized five-grass-pollen extract (drops and sublingual tablets) versus placebo in seasonal rhinitis. Allergy 1999;54:819–828.

10   Seibel K, Schaffler K, Reitmeir P: A randomised, placebo-controlled study comparing two formulations of dimenhydrinate with respect to efficacy in motion sickness and sedation. Arzneimittelforschung 2002;52:529–536.

11   Wozniak KL, Arribas A, Leigh JE, Fidel PL Jr: Inhibitory effects of whole and parotid saliva on immunomodulators. Oral Microbiol Immunol 2002;17:100–107.

12   Walker GF, Langoth N, Bernkop-Schnurch A: Peptidase activity on the surface of the porcine buccal mucosa. Int J Pharm 2002;233:141–147.

13   Gelfand EW, Cui ZH, Takeda K, Kanehiro A, Joetham A: Fexofenadine modulates T-cell function, preventing allergen-induced airway inflammation and hyperresponsiveness. J Allergy Clin Immunol 2002;110:85–95.

14   Kuehr J, Brauburger J, Zielen S, Schauer U, Kamin W, Von Berg A, Leupold W, Bergmann KC, Rolinck-Werninghaus C, Grave M, Hultsch T, Wahn U: Efficacy of combination treatment with anti-IgE plus specific immunotherapy in polysensitized children and adolescents with seasonal allergic rhinitis. J Allergy Clin Immunol 2002;109:274–280.

15   Andre C, Vatrinet C, Galvain S, Carat F, Sicard H: Safety of sublingual-swallow immunotherapy in children and adults. Int Arch Allergy Immunol 2000;121:229–234.

16   Voltolini S, Modena P, Minale P, Bignardi D, Troise C, Puccinelli P, Parmiani S: Sublingual immunotherapy in tree pollen allergy. Double-blind, placebo-controlled study with a biologically standardised extract of three pollens (alder, birch and hazel) administered by a rush schedule. Allergol Immunopathol 2001;29:103–110.

17   Moller C, Dreborg S, Ferdousi HA, Halken S, Host A, Jacobsen L, Koivikko A, Koller DY, Niggemann B, Norberg LA, Urbanek R, Valovirta E, Wahn U: Pollen immunotherapy reduces the development of asthma in children with seasonal rhinoconjunctivitis (the PAT-study). J Allergy Clin Immunol 2002;109:251–256.

18   Passalacqua G, Albano M, Fregonese L, Riccio A, Pronzato C, Mela GS, Canonica GW: Randomised controlled trial of local allergoid immunotherapy on allergic inflammation in mite-induced rhinoconjunctivitis. Lancet 1998;351:629–632.

19   Bagnasco M, Passalacqua G, Villa G, Augeri C, Flamigni G, Borini E, Falagiani P, Mistrello G, Canonica GW, Mariani G: Pharmacokinetics of an allergen and a monomeric allergoid for oro-mucosal immunotherapy in allergic volunteers. Clin Exp Allergy 2001;31:54–60.

20   Herz U, Joachim R, Ahrens B, Scheffold A, Radbruch A, Renz H: Allergic sensitization and allergen exposure during pregnancy favor the development of atopy in the neonate. Int Arch Allergy Immunol 2001;124:193–196.

21   Purello-D'Ambrosio F, Gangemi S, Merendino RA, Isola S, Puccinelli P, Parmiani S, Ricciardi L: Prevention of new sensitizations in monosensitized subjects submitted to specific immunotherapy or not. A retrospective study. Clin Exp Allergy 2001;31:1295–1302.

22   Bousquet J, Demoly P, Michel FB: Specific immunotherapy in rhinitis and asthma. Ann Allergy Asthma Immunol 2001;87(suppl 1):38–42.

23   Mastrandrea F, Serio G, Minelli M, Minardi A, Scarcia G, Coradduzza G, Parmiani S: Specific sublingual immunotherapy in atopic dermatitis. Results of a 6-year follow-up of 35 consecutive patients. Allergol Immunopathol 2000;28:54–62.

24   Shaikh WA: A retrospective study on the safety of immunotherapy in pregnancy. Clin Exp Allergy 1993;23:857–860.

25 Mazzotta P, Loebstein R, Koren G: Treating allergic rhinitis in pregnancy. Safety considerations. Drug Saf 1999;20:361–375.

26 Schatz M, Zeiger RS: Asthma and allergy in pregnancy. Clin Perinatol 1997;24:407–432.

27 Passalacqua G, Fumagalli F, Guerra L, Canonica GW: Safety of allergen-specific sublingual immunotherapy and nasal immunotherapy. Chem Immunol Allergy. Basel, Karger, 2003, vol 82, pp 109–118.

28 Horak F, Stubner P, Berger UE, Marks B, Toth J, Jager S: Immunotherapy with sublingual birch pollen extract. A short-term double-blind placebo study. J Investig Allergol Clin Immunol 1998;8: 165–171.

29 Mungan D, Misirligil Z, Gurbuz L: Comparison of the efficacy of subcutaneous and sublingual immunotherapy in mite-sensitive patients with rhinitis and asthma – A placebo controlled study. Ann Allergy Asthma Immunol 1999;82:485–490.

30 Quirino T, Iemoli E, Siciliani E, Parmiani S, Milazzo F: Sublingual versus injective immunotherapy in grass pollen allergic patients: A double blind (double dummy) study. Clin Exp Allergy 1996;26:1253–1261.

31 Guez S: Efficacy of desensitization via the sublingual route in mite allergy. Chem Immunol Allergy. Basel, Karger, 2003, vol 82, pp 62–76.

Dr. Udo R. Markert
Abteilung für Geburtshilfe, Friedrich-Schiller-Universität,
D–07740 Jena (Germany)
Tel. +49 3641 933763, Fax +49 3641 933764 E-Mail udo.markert@med.uni-jena.de

Author Index

Subject Index